Glucagon in 1987

Glucagon in 1987

Gastrointestinal and Hepatobiliary Physiology, Diagnosis and Treatment

EDITED BY

J. Picazo, MD

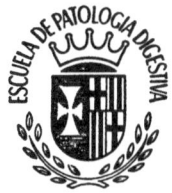

*Proceedings of an International Workshop
held in Barcelona on 6 March 1987,
under the auspices of the Escuela de Patología Digestiva
of the Universidad Autónoma, Barcelona*

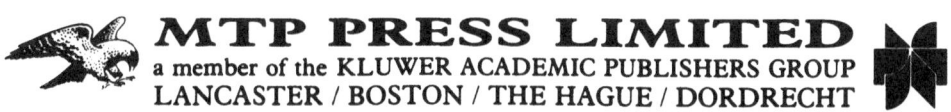

MTP PRESS LIMITED
a member of the KLUWER ACADEMIC PUBLISHERS GROUP
LANCASTER / BOSTON / THE HAGUE / DORDRECHT

Published in the UK and Europe by
MTP Press Limited
Falcon House
Lancaster, England

British Library Cataloguing in Publication Data

Glucagon in 1987: gastrointestinal and hepatobiliary physiology, diagnosis and treatment:
proceedings of an international workshop held in Barcelona on 6 March 1987, under the
auspices of the Escuela de Patologia Digestiva of the Universidad Autonoma, Barcelona.
1. Gastroenterology   2. Glucagon
I. Picazo, J.   II. Universidad Autonoma, Barcelona. *Escuela de Patologia Digestiva*
616.3'3   RC817

ISBN-13: 978-94-010-7929-7   e-ISBN-13: 978-94-009-3185-5
DOI: 10.1007/978-94-009-3185-5

Published in the USA by
MTP Press
A division of Kluwer Academic Publishers
101 Philip Drive
Norwell, MA 02061, USA

Contents

List of Participants   vii

Preface
F. Vilardell   ix

GASTROENTEROLOGY SESSION

1 Accumulated experience in the physiology of glucagon
   P.J. Lefèbvre   3

2 Effect of glucagon on haemodynamics and gastrointestinal tract
   motility. Role of the glucagon receptor
   L. Santamaría and E. De Miguel   15

3 Glucagon in upper gastrointestinal radiology
   M. Maruyama   29

4 Lower gastrointestinal tract radiology with glucagon
   J. Skucas   41

5 Glucagon in digestive endoscopy – its usefulness for premedication
   *T. Takemoto, K. Okita, T. Tada, H. Kawano, T. Yoshida and
   T. Akiyama*   55

6 Glucagon and the human biliary tree
   D.L. Carr-Locke   67

   General discussion
   Chairmen: A. Oriol-Bosch and F. Vilardell   87

HEPATOLOGY SESSION

7   Experimental evidence of the hepatotrophic effect of insulin and glucagon
    K. Fujiwara, I. Ogata, S. Mishiro, Y. Ohta, Y. Oka, K. Takatsuki, Y. Sato, S. Hayashi, S. Yamada and H. Oka   99

8   Insulin and glucagon infusion therapy in acute alcoholic hepatitis
    J. Fehér, A. Cornides, A. Gógl, A. Romány, M. Kartészi, L. Szalay and J. Picazo   111

9   Clinical evaluation of glucagon-insulin therapy for acute hepatitis severe form
    H. Oka, K. Fujiwara, K. Okita, H. Ishii and A. Sakuma   125

10 Clinical evaluation of glucagon and insulin in therapy of fulminant hepatitis
    K. Okita, S. Matsuda and T. Takemoto   135

11 A clinical perspective on hepatic regeneration
    A. L. Baker   147

    General discussion
    Chairmen: A. Oriol-Bosch and F. Vilardell   161

    Remarks from the chairmen   167

    Index   169

List of Participants

A. L. BAKER
Liver Study Unit
University of Chicago
Chicago, IL 60637
USA

D. L. CARR-LOCKE
The Leicester Royal Infirmary
Leicester, LE1 5WW
UK

E. DE MIGUEL
Department of Experimental Surgery
La Paz Medical Center
Madrid
Spain

J. FEHÉR
Second Department of Medicine
Semmelweis University
H-1088 Budapest
Hungary

K. FUJIWARA
First Department of Internal Medicine
University of Tokyo
Tokyo 113
Japan

P. J. LEFÈBVRE
Institute of Medicine
Hôpital de Bavière
B-4020 Liege
Belgium

M. MARUYAMA
Department of Internal Medicine
Cancer Institute Hospital
Tokyo
Japan

S. MATSUDA
Department of Gastroenterology
National Shimonoseki Hospital
Shimonoseki, Yamaguchi 751
Japan

N. A. NIKOLOV
Department of Pathophysiology
Medical Academy
BG-1431 Sofia
Bulgaria

H. OKA
First Department of Internal Medicine
University of Tokyo
Tokyo 113
Japan

K. OKITA
First Department of Internal Medicine
University of Yamaguchi
Ube, Yamaguchi 755
Japan

A. ORIOL-BOSCH
Department of Experimental Endocrinology
Facultad de Medicina,
Universidad Complutense
28003 Madrid
Spain

L. SANTAMARÍA
Department of Morphology
Facultad de Medicina,
Universidad Autónoma
28040 Madrid
Spain

J. SKUCAS
Department of Radiology
Rochester University Medical Center
Rochester, NY 14642
USA

T. TAKEMOTO
First Department of Internal Medicine
University of Yamaguchi
Ube, Yamaguchi 755
Japan

F. VILARDELL
Escuela de Patología Digestiva
Universidad Autónoma
08025 Barcelona
Spain

Preface

I am very pleased to say once again that I was delighted at being invited to chair this Third International Workshop on Glucagon (*Glucagon in 1987*). The two previous ones were held in Madrid under the auspices of the Medical School of the Universidad Complutense of that city, the first in May 1978 and the second in October 1981, which resulted in two books (*Glucagon in Gastroenterology*, 1979, and *Glucagon in Gastroenterology and Hepatology*, 1982, both published by MTP Press), where the mounting interest in and developments concerning the therapeutic applications of glucagon were reflected. This time the meeting was held in Barcelona under the auspices of the Escuela de Patología Digestiva of the Universidad Autónoma of Barcelona, a change that we especially welcomed because it is not very often that we are able to assemble in our city such a distinguished group of scientists from all over the world. As can be seen from the title of the present book, this workshop focussed once again on the current status of glucagon in gastroenterology and hepatology, because although much has been said and discussed about the subject already, it still raises exciting and intriguing issues for debate.

There were two parts to this meeting. The gastroenterology session was concerned with the physiology and pathophysiology of glucagon in the gastrointestinal tract and its applications in diagnosis, endoscopy and radiology. The biliary tree was also discussed in depth since this topic continues to be of potential future interest. The second session was devoted to the liver, a subject that is gathering momentum year by year.

The format of this workshop was very much the same as that of the previous ones, with a small group of international multidisciplinary participants assembled for a one-day work event to cover as widely as possible one specific topic from all its perspectives. This book is the result of that day of work and in it are the papers that were presented and the edited version of the discussions.

Two exceptions were made to the usual arrangements. In the first place, Professor Lefèbvre was unfortunately unable to attend the whole meeting, but I would like to express my appreciation to him, which I am sure will be shared by everyone involved, for his kindness in contributing a very informative paper and providing very interesting discussion topics during some brief hours which he literally squeezed into his tight schedule. It is for this reason that the General Discussion was divided into a morning session and an afternoon session, in order to have Professor Lefèbvre's valuable contribution at least in one of them. Another exception is the publication in this book of a paper by Dr L. Santamaría, who in the end was unable to be with us at the workshop. Nonetheless, it was considered that the information he should have presented merited inclusion even if it was not discussed at the meeting. Such exceptions are almost unavoidable for workshops like this when important people from all over the world must be assembled on one particular day.

I had the chance to thank all the participants at the workshop, but I would like to take this opportunity to thank them again most heartily for their contributions and cooperation, not only during the meeting, but also before and after it, for without them it would not have been possible to present and to disseminate so much information, nor would this book exist. I also extend my thanks to Dr José Picazo who organized the event and made it possible for all of us to meet, and I congratulate him, Mari Carmen Hernández and María Picazo on the publication of this book, for it was they who had to gather the manuscripts together and pull our far-ranging discussions into shape. Finally, I would like to thank our publishers for working so cooperatively to produce this book. In short, to everyone involved I extend my thanks for your contributions to what I feel to be a most interesting and worthwhile project.

Barcelona
October 1987

F. Vilardell

Gastroenterology Session

1
Accumulated experience in the physiology of glucagon

P. J. LEFÈBVRE

INTRODUCTION

Before being a useful spasmolytic and hepatotrophic drug, glucagon is an important hormone exerting major metabolic effects in animals and in man. The explosion of our knowledge of glucagon is reflected by the size of some of the monographs and books devoted to glucagon and published over the last 30 years (Figure 1.1). The last comprehensive book on glucagon was published in 1983, and consists of two volumes totalling 1235 pages[1]. Most of the data summarized hereafter are developed in detail in the 56 chapters of these volumes.

STRUCTURE AND BIOSYNTHESIS OF GLUCAGON

As reviewed by Bromer[2], the amino-acid sequence is identical for glucagon isolated from the pancreas of pigs, cattle, and humans. Guinea-pig glucagon is quite different from all other glucagons that have been isolated while avian glucagons differ from the predominant mammalian glucagon by only a few conservative replacements. This extreme conservation of the primary structure exhibited by glucagon 'can at least be termed unusual and, at most, extra-ordinary'[2]. Mammalian glucagon contains 29 amino-acid residues and has a molecular weight of 3485 daltons (Figure 1.2). Glucagon can be synthe-sized *in vitro* by either classical solution synthesis or solid phase synthesis; in both cases, two sub-strategies can be used, either fragment assembly or

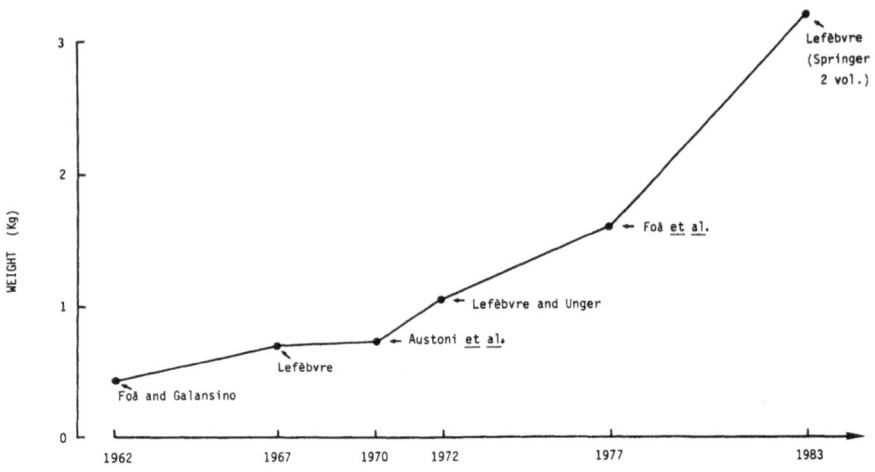

Figure 1.1   Weight of books on glucagon published over the last 25 years[1, 38–42]

H–HIS–SER–GLN–GLY–THR–PHE–THR–SER–ASP–TYR–SER–LYS–TYR–LEU–ASP–
 1   2   3   4   5   6   7   8   9   10   11   12   13   14   15

SER–ARG–ARG–ALA–GLN–ASP–PHE–VAL–GLN–TRP–LEU–MET–ASN–THR–OH
16   17   18   19   20   21   22   23   24   25   26   27   28   29

Figure 1.2   The primary structure of mammalian glucagon

stepwise assembly (as reviewed by Merrifield and Mojsov[3]). All procedures have resulted in highly purified materials that are homogeneous and indistinguishable from natural glucagon according to a range of sensitive analytic methods.

Naturally occurring glucagon originates in the A-cells of the islets of Langerhans of the pancreas. In addition, in some species like the dog or the rat, glucagon is also synthesized in 'true A-cells' located in the fundus of the stomach. The presence of extrapancreatic A-cells in the adult human stomach is still a matter of controversy[4, 5]. As reviewed by Hellerström[6], there is now agreement that glucagon is synthesized via a larger precursor, which is processed towards glucagon through a stepwise proteolytic degradation. Although the size of preproglucagon is still a matter of controversy, there is little doubt that an intermediate, proglucagon (most probably identical to

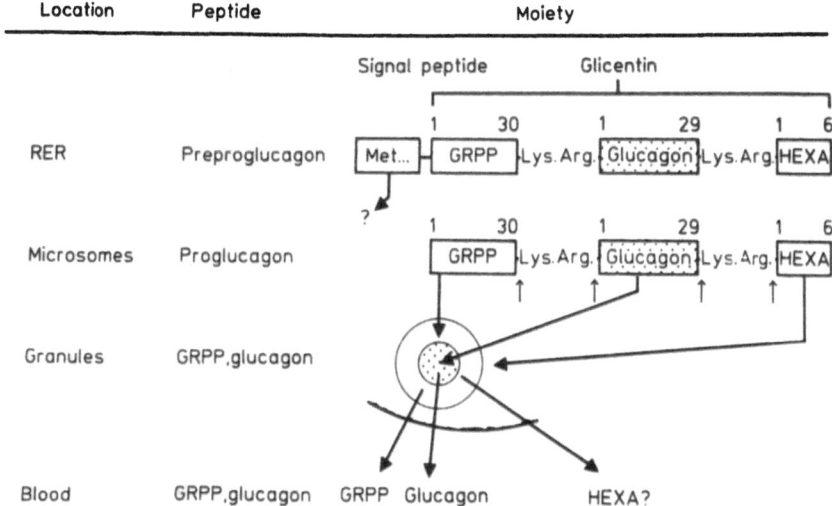

Figure 1.3 A proposed conversion of porcine proglucagon (identical to glicentin) into glucagon, GRPP (glicentin-related pancreatic peptide) and hexapeptide (HEXA). RER = rough endoplasmic reticulum

glicentin)[7], is stored together with glucagon itself in the secretory granules of the pancreatic A-cells and is secreted along with the native hormone (Figure 1.3).

Glicentin (or proglucagon) is converted into glucagon (29 amino-acid residues), a glicentin-related pancreatic peptide (GRPP) with 30 amino-acid residues, and a hexapeptide (corresponding to the last six amino-acids of the glicentin molecule). Another peptide has also been isolated: it corresponds to glucagon extended at the carboxyl terminal by the carboxyl terminal octopeptide of glicentin, it is therefore identical to glicentin 33–69 and has been termed oxyntomodulin[8].

Glicentin is also produced by the L-cells of the intestine and probably constitutes a major part of the so-called 'gut glucagon-like immunoreactive materials'[7]. The observation that glicentin is stored in the secretory granules of those cells without being converted to glucagon requires further studies. Data from Korànyi et al.[9] have suggested that some glucagon might be generated from glicentin in the circulating blood. According to Moody and Thim[7], the roles of glicentin and other gut glucagon-like immunoreactive substances (GLIs) in the whole organism remain to be established. There are grounds for proposing that the primary target organs of the gut GLIs are in the gastroenteropancreatic system, as inducers of the system's post-natal development and maturation and, possibly, as weak glucagon agonists'[7].

Data from Bataille and his coworkers[10] have convincingly demonstrated the existence of specific sites for oxyntomodulin in isolated oxyntic glands from rat fundic mucosa. The possibility that this substance may play a role in inhibiting gastric acid secretion has been raised[11].

PHYSIOLOGICAL ACTIONS OF GLUCAGON

Glucagon acts by binding to specific receptors located at the target cell plasma membranes. The major common effect of glucagon is to activate adenylate (also called adenylyl cyclase) and to increase the intracellular production of cyclic AMP. Rodbell[12] has reported that there is now considerable evidence that the binding of glucagon to its receptor activates an intermediate transduction process which involves the participation of GTP, divalent cations and adenosine (or other similar natural substances). The hepatocyte is a major target cell of glucagon. The main effect of glucagon on the liver is to increase glucose output, an effect which results from the inhibition of glycogen synthesis, stimulation of liver glycogenolysis and gluconeogenesis. Stalmans[13] and Claus et al.[14] report on the mechanism involved with more detail. There is ample evidence that most of these effects are mediated by cyclic AMP but the possibility has been raised that part of the glycogenolytic effect of glucagon may occur by a cAMP-independent mechanism, the nature of which has not been established yet[13]. Another major effect of glucagon on the liver is to stimulate ketogenesis. The elegant studies of McGarry and Foster[15] have convincingly shown that liver ketogenesis depends on both the flux of free fatty acids (FFA) into the liver and on the enzymatic setting of this organ, which is influenced in a crucial manner by the glucagon/insulin ratio in the blood perfusing the liver. These authors have shown that a high glucagon/insulin ratio increases the intracellular level of cAMP, reduces glycogenolysis and acetyl-CoA carboxylase activity, and reduces the intracellular concentration of malonyl-CoA. This fall in malonyl-CoA brings fatty acid synthesis to a halt and causes derepression of the enzyme carnitine acyltransferase in such a way that incoming fatty acids (made abundant through stimulation of lipolysis) are efficiently converted into the ketone bodies, acetoacetate and β-hydroxybutyrate. The effects of glucagon on the adipocyte are highly dependent upon the species considered. While glucagon is a potent lipolytic hormone in birds and in rodents, its effects on the human adipose cell have been disputed[16]. Recent investigations have shown that indeed glucagon is strongly lipolytic in the human adipocyte in vitro but that this effect is difficult to demonstrate using incubation of adipose cells or adipose tissue pieces because glucagon is rapidly destroyed by a proteolytic activity associated with those cells[17]. When perfusion techniques are used, the lipolytic effect of glucagon on human adipocytes can easily be demonstrated[17]. All those effects of glucagon (stimulation of liver glucose output, hepatic ketogenesis and adipose tissue lipolysis) qualify it as a 'hormone of energy need'[18] as will be discussed later.

OTHER EFFECTS OF GLUCAGON

Other metabolic effects of glucagon include the modification of the circulatory pattern of plasma amino acids (partly due to the stimulation of gluconeogenesis) and a reduction in cholesterol and triglyceride circulating levels[19]. Glucagon also stimulates insulin release[20, 21]. It plays a major role, together with insulin, in liver regeneration[22]. Under certain circumstances, glucagon increases renal blood flow and glomerular filtration rate, and promotes renal loss of sodium and other ions[23]. At pharmacological doses, glucagon stimulates adrenal catecholamine release, an effect which has been used for the diagnosis of phaeochromocytoma[24]. Farah[25] has shown that glucagon also exerts positive inotropic and chronotropic effects on the heart, effects that might be useful, for instance, in treating the cardiodepressive manifestations of β-receptor blocking agent poisoning; glucagon and several of its analogues (like glucagon 1–21-peptide which is devoid of metabolic effects) exert a potent smooth muscle spasmolytic action largely used for various diagnostic procedures or for therapeutic applications[26], as will be discussed in detail in other chapters of this book.

CONTROL OF GLUCAGON RELEASE

Table 1.1 lists the factors and conditions demonstrated to stimulate glucagon

Table 1.1   Stimulants of glucagon release

Substrates:	Hypoglycaemia or cytoglycopenia (2-deoxy-glucose) Low circulating levels of free fatty acids Most amino-acids Fumarate and glutamate
Neural factors:	Stimulation of adrenergic and cholinergic nervous systems Stimulation of ventromedial (and ventrolateral?) hypothalamus
Local transmitters or factors:	Adrenaline, noradrenaline, acetylcholine, dopamine, vasoactive intestinal peptide (VIP), neurotensin, bombesin, substance P, prostaglandins, AMP, β-endorphin
Hormones:	Gastrin, cholecystokinin–pancreozymin (CCK-PZ), gastric inhibitory peptide (GIP), growth hormone
Ions:	Total absence of calcium Lack of phosphate or of magnesium Potassium (?)
Pharmacological agents:	Furosemide, scorpion venom, phospholipase A2, L-DOPA
Situations:	Starvation, exercise, stress, balanced meal

secretion. The main physiological or pathophysiological stimulators of glucagon release are hypoglycaemia (insulin-induced, associated with starvation or intense muscular exercise), hyperaminoacidaemia (the rise in plasma glucagon levels after a balanced meal is probably due mainly to amino-acid-induced glucagon release), stimulation of the adrenergic system (stress, exercise), and stimulation of the vagal system (which together with hormones like gastric inhibitory peptide and cholecystokinin–pancreozymin probably participate in the mixed meal-induced glucagon rise).

The factors and conditions associated with an inhibition of glucagon release are listed in Table 1.2. The main physiological inhibitors of glucagon release are probably hyperglycaemia and hyperinsulinaemia (in a glucose- or carbohydrate-rich meal) and high circulating levels of FFA. The pharmacological inhibition of glucagon release may participate in various drug-induced hypoglycaemic syndromes.

Table 1.2 Inhibitors of glucagon release

Substrates:	Hyperglycaemia (also fructose and xylitol) High circulating levels of FFA (and ketone bodies)
Local transmitters or factors:	Serotonin, somatostatin
Hormones:	Insulin, secretin, oestrogens
Ions:	Calcium, magnesium
Pharmacological agents:	Atropine, β-receptor blocking agents, indomethacin, meclofenamate, ibuprofen, diphenylhydantoin, procaine, diazepam, phenformin, various somatostatin analogues, diazoxide (?), sulphonylureas (?)
Situations:	Carbohydrate meal, pregnancy

Samols and his coworkers[27] have emphasized the delicate mechanisms by which intra-islet insulin, glucagon and somatostatin release may be interrelated. In those paracrine mechanisms, recent data have suggested that the oscillatory pattern of islet hormone release may be particularly important[28].

SOME ASPECTS OF GLUCAGON PHYSIOLOGY

Glucagon as a counter-regulatory hormone

Numerous recent studies, reviewed by Gerich[29] and Lickley et al.[30], have shown that 'the liver is the main site at which moment-to-moment control of glucose homeostasis takes place and that in normal humans glucagon is the major glucose counter-regulatory hormone; by antagonizing the suppressive effects of insulin on glucose production and by stimulating glucose production when appropriate, glucagon not only defends the organism against hypoglycaemia, but also restores normoglycaemia if hypoglycaemia occurs'[29]. Perturbation of the mechanisms controlling hypoglycaemia-induced glucagon release in some diabetic patients markedly increases the risk of severe hypoglycaemia in these subjects[31]. Other hormones, like epinephrine, acutely, and growth hormone and cortisol, more slowly, participate in the counter-regulation of the effects of insulin, but careful clinical observations suggest that indeed glucagon is the *first line of defence* against hypoglycaemia[32].

Glucagon in exercise

Glucagon levels increase progressively during prolonged duration exercise[33], a condition during which blood glucose remains relatively constant thanks to a fine balance between muscle glucose uptake and liver glucose production. Although a rise in plasma glucagon does not appear to be essential for increased glucagon production during exercise, the presence of glucagon does appear to be necessary[30].

Glucagon in stress

Hyperglucagonaemia is a classical feature of stress[34]. It occurs mainly as a result of the β-adrenergic stimulation associated with stress[30] and undoubtedly contributes to the hyperglycaemia classically observed in this condition.

Glucagon in starvation

Starvation is accompanied by a decline in circulating insulin and a moderate rise in plasma glucagon[35]. The main effects of glucagon during starvation are at the liver site where it contributes to the maintenance of continuous liver glucose output (initially by stimulating glycogenolysis, later by promoting glyconeogenesis) and inducing ketogenesis[36]. A contribution of glucagon in stimulating adipose tissue lipolysis during starvation has been disputed, but recent observations made on human perfused adipocytes make it plausible[17].

Glucagon and adaptation to extra-uterine life

A significant rise in plasma glucagon occurs soon after birth in all the species investigated so far[37] and suggests that glucagon plays a crucial role in neonatal glucose homeostasis.

CONCLUSIONS

In addition to being a useful pharmacological agent because of its spasmolytic and hepatotrophic properties, glucagon is an important hormone which exerts numerous metabolic actions including stimulation of hepatic glycogenolysis and gluconeogenesis, inhibition of liver glycogen synthesis, stimulation of adipose tissue lipolysis and of hepatic ketogenesis. All these effects of glucagon are strongly antagonized by insulin. Glucagon originates from the A-cells of the islets of Langerhans of the pancreas where it is synthesized in the form of a large precursor, identical to glicentin, one of the components of gut 'glucagon-like' immunoreactivity (GLI). Glucagon release is stimulated in various physiological situations including hypoglycaemia, low circulating levels of free fatty acids, high levels of numerous amino-acids, stimulation of both vagal and adrenergic nervous system, etc. Prolonged starvation, long-duration exercise and adaptation to extra-uterine life are also associated with high circulating levels of glucagon. All these effects of glucagon make it, *par excellence*, a hormone of energy need.

References

1. Lefèbvre PJ. *Glucagon. Handb Exp Pharmacol 66 I and II.* Berlin, Heidelberg, New York, Tokyo: Springer, 1983.
2. Bromer WW. Chemical characteristics of glucagon. In: Lefèbvre PJ, ed. *Glucagon I. Handb Exp Pharmacol 66 I.* Berlin, Heidelberg, New York, Tokyo: Springer, 1983: 1–22.
3. Merrifield RB, Mojsov S. The chemical synthesis of glucagon. In: Lefèbvre PJ, ed. *Glucagon I. Handb Exp Pharmacol 66 I.* Berlin, Heidelberg, New York, Tokyo: Springer, 1983: 23–25.
4. Orci L, Bordi C, Unger RH, Perrelet A. Glucagon- and glicentin-producing cells. In: Lefèbvre PJ, ed. *Glucagon I. Handb Exp Pharmacol 66 I.* Berlin, Heidelberg, New York, Tokyo: Springer, 1983: 57–79.
5. Lefèbvre PJ, Luyckx AS. Extrapancreatic glucagon and its regulation. In: Lefèbvre PJ, ed. *Glucagon II. Handb Exp Pharmacol 66 II* Berlin, Heidelberg, New York, Tokyo: Springer, 1983: 205–219.
6. Hellerström C. Biosynthesis of glucagon. In: Lefèbvre PJ, ed. *Glucagon I. Handb Exp Pharmacol 66 I.* Berlin, Heidelberg, New York, Tokyo: Springer, 1983: 121–138.
7. Moody AJ, Thim L. Glucagon, glicentin and related peptides. In: Lefèbvre PJ, ed. *Glucagon I. Handb Exp Pharmacol 66 I.* Berlin, Heidelberg, New York, Tokyo: Springer, 1983: 139–174.
8. Bataille D, Gespach C, Tatemoto K, Marie JC, Caudray AM, Rosselin G, Mutt V. Bioactive enteroglucagon (oxyntomodulin): Present knowledge of its chemical structure and its biological activities. *Peptides* 1981; 2 (suppl 2): 41–44.
9. Korànyi L, Peterfy, F, Szabo J, Török A, Guoth M, Tamas GY Jr. Evidence for transformation of glucagon-like immunoreactivity of gut into pancreatic glucagon *in vivo. Diabetes* 1981; 30: 792–794.
10. Bataille D, Tatemoto K, Gespach H, Jornvall H, Rosselin G, Mutt V. Isolation of glucagon-37 (bioactive enteroglucagon/oxyntomodulin) from porcine jejuno-ileum. Characterization of the peptide. *FEBS Lett* 1982; 146: 79–86.
11. Depigny C, Lupo B, Kervran A, Bataille D. Mise en évidence d'un site récepteur spécifique du glucagon 37 (oxyntomoduline/entero-glucagon bioactif) dans les glandes oxyntiques du rat. *CR Acad Sci (Paris)* 1984; 299: 677–680.
12. Rodbell M. The actions of glucagon at its receptor: regulation of adenylate cyclase. In:

ACCUMULATED EXPERIENCE IN THE PHYSIOLOGY OF GLUCAGON

Lefèbvre PJ, ed. *Glucagon I. Handb Exp Pharmacol 66 I.* Berlin, Heidelberg, New York, Tokyo: Springer, 1983: 263–290.

13. Stalmans W. Glucagon and liver glycogen metabolism. In: Lefèbvre PJ, ed. *Glucagon I. Handb Exp Pharmacol 66 I.* Berlin, Heidelberg, New York, Tokyo: Springer, 1983: 291–314.

14. Claus TH, Park CR, Pilkis SJ. Glucagon and gluconeogenesis. In: Lefèbvre PJ, ed. *Glucagon I. Handb Exp Pharmacol 66 I.* Berlin, Heidelberg, New York, Tokyo: Springer, 1983: 315–360.

15. McGarry JD, Foster DW. Glucagon and ketogenesis. In: Lefèbvre PJ, ed. *Glucagon I. Handb Exp Pharmacol 66 I.* Berlin, Heidelberg, New York, Tokyo: Springer, 1983: 383–389.

16. Lefèbvre PJ. Glucagon and adipose tissue lipolysis. In: Lefèbvre PJ, ed. *Glucagon I. Handb Exp Pharmacol 66 I.* Berlin, Heidelberg, New York, Tokyo: Springer, 1983: 419–440.

17. Korànyi L. Lipolytic effect of glucagon on perfused isolated human fat cells. *Diabetologia* 1983; 25: 172.

18. Lefèbvre PJ. Commentary: Glucagon and adipose tissue. *Biochem Pharmacol* 1975; 24: 1261–1266.

19. Tiengo A, Nosadini R. Glucagon and lipoprotein metabolism. In: Lefèbvre PJ, ed. *Glucagon I. Handb Exp Pharmacol 66 I.* Berlin, Heidelberg, New York, Tokyo: Springer, 1983: 441–451.

20. Samols E, Marri G, Marks V. Promotion of insulin secretion by glucagon. *Lancet* 1965: 2: 415–416.

21. Samols E. Glucagon and insulin secretion. In: Lefèbvre PJ, ed. *Glucagon I. Handb Exp Pharmacol 66 I.* Berlin, Heidelberg, New York, Tokyo: Springer, 1983: 485–518.

22. Leffert HL, Koch KS, Lad PJ, De Hemptinne B, Skelly H. Glucagon and liver regeneration. In: Lefèbvre PJ, ed. *Glucagon I. Handb Exp Pharmacol 66 I.* Berlin, Heidelberg, New York, Tokyo: Springer, 1983: 453–484.

23. Kolanowski J. Influence of glucagon on water and electrolyte metabolism. In: Lefèbvre PJ, ed. *Glucagon II. Handb Exp Pharmacol 66 II.* Berlin, Heidelberg, New York, Tokyo: Springer, 1983: 525–536.

24. Lefèbvre PJ, Luyckx AS. Glucagon and catecholamines. In: Lefèbvre PJ, ed. *Glucagon II. Handb Exp Pharmacol 66 II.* Berlin, Heidelberg, New York, Tokyo: Springer, 1983: 537–543.

25. Farah AH. Glucagon and the heart. In: Lefèbvre PJ, ed. *Glucagon II. Handb Exp Pharmacol 66 I.* Berlin, Heidelberg, New York, Tokyo: Springer, 1983: 553–609.

26. Diamant D, Picazo J. Spasmolytic action and clinical use of glucagon. In: Lefèbvre PJ, ed. *Glucagon II. Handb Exp Pharmacol 66 II.* Berlin, Heidelberg, New York, Tokyo: Springer, 1983: 611–643.

27. Samols E, Weir GC, Bonner-Weir S. Intra-islet insulin-glucagon-somatostatin relationships. In: Lefèbvre PJ, ed. *Glucagon II. Handb Exp Pharmacol 66 II.* Berlin, Heidelberg, New York, Tokyo: Springer, 1983: 133–173.

28. Paolisso G, Sgambato S, Passariello N, Varrichio M. Scheen A, D'Onofrio F, Lefèbvre PJ. Pulsatile insulin delivery is more efficient than continuous infusion in modulating islet-cell function in normal subjects and in patients with type-1 diabetes. (Submitted for publication.)

29. Gerich JE. Glucagon as a counter-regulatory hormone. In: Lefèbvre PJ, ed. *Glucagon II. Handb Exp Pharmacol 66 II.* Berlin, Heidelberg, New York, Tokyo: Springer, 1983: 275–295.

30. Lickley HLA, Kemmer FW, Wasserman DH, Vranic M. Glucagon and its relationship to other glucoregulatory hormones in exercise and stress in normal and diabetic subjects. In: Lefèbvre PJ, ed. *Glucagon II. Handb Exp Pharmacol 66 II.* Berlin, Heidelberg, New York, Tokyo: Springer, 1983: 297–350.

31. White NH, Skor DA, Cryer PE, Levandorsky LA, Bier DM. Identification of type-1 diabetic patients at increased risk for hypoglycemia during intensive therapy. *N. Engl J Med* 1983; 308: 485–491.

32. Gerich J, Davis J, Lorenzi M, Rizza R, Karam J, Lewis S, Kaplan R, Schultz T, Cryer P. Hormonal mechanisms of recovery from insulin-induced hypoglycemia in man. *Am J Physiol* 1979; 236: 380–385.

33. Luyckx AS, Pirnay F, Lefèbvre PJ. Effect of glucose on plasma glucagon and free fatty acids during prolonged exercise. *Eur J Appl Physiol* 1978; 39: 53–61.
34. Lindsey CA, Faloona GR, Unger RH. Plasma glucagon levels during rapid exsanguination with and without adrenergic blockade. *Diabetes* 1975; 24: 313–319.
35. Cahill GF Jr. Starvation in man. *N Engl J Med* 1970; 282: 668–675.
36. Gelfand RA, Sherwin RS. Glucagon and starvation. In: Lefèbvre PJ, ed. *Glucagon II. Handb Exp Pharmacol 66 II* Berlin, Heidelberg, New York, Tokyo: Springer, 1983: 223–237.
37. Girard J, Sperling M. Glucagon in the fetus and the newborn. In: Lefèbvre PJ, ed. *Glucagon II. Handb Exp Pharmacol 66 II.* Berlin, Heidelberg, New York, Tokyo: Springer, 1983: 251–274.
38. Foà PP. Galansino G. *Glucagon. Chemistry and Function in Health and Disease.* Springfield: CC Thomas, 1962.
39. Lefèbvre P. *Le Glucagon, Seconde Hormone Pancréatique.* Paris: Maloine, 1967.
40. Austoni M, Scandellari C, Federspil G, Trisotto A. *Current Topics on Glucagon.* Padova: CEDAM, 1971.
41. Lefébvre PJ, Unger RH. *Glucagon. Molecular Physiology, Clinical and Therapeutic Implications.* Oxford: Pergamon Press, 1972.
42. Foà PP, Bajaj JS, Foà NL. *Glucagon: Its Role in Physiology and Clinical Medicine.* New York, Heidelberg, Berlin: Springer, 1977.

DISCUSSION

Nikolov Professor Lefèbvre, you have mentioned antibodies. Have you had any experience in which glucagon secretion has been inhibited by antibodies? Because, to my knowledge, glucagon shows a very low antigenicity. Do you have some personal experience in this field?

Lefèbvre No, I am afraid I do not.

Nikolov Do you know of any receptor blocking agent which can block specifically the effect of glucagon on cyclic AMP?

Lefèbvre Well, there has been a compound, dehistidine glucagon as a matter of fact, a glucagon from which histidine has been removed, which has been shown to act that way (Bromer WW. *Metabolism* 1976; (Suppl) 25: 1315–1316).

Nikolov But we know that these receptors for B effects are mediated by many different hormones. ...

Lefèbvre Yes, that is right.

Nikolov Could you comment further on the specific actions of glucagon on cyclic AMP?

Lefèbvre I think we should start off from the basis that in all circumstances, almost all the effects of glucagon can also be produced by other compounds, such as epinephrine for instance. The real problem is raised by the fine analysis of the things occurring under physiological conditions, in order to see which of them is interfering. Actually, we did this some years ago and we reached the conclusion that in the case of exercise, for example, glucagon is probably a major operating hormone, but if we suppress glucagon by pharmacological means, the effects will still be present, because there are other hormones which come to replace glucagon (Lefèbvre PJ *Biochem Pharmacol* 1975; 24: 1261–1266).

Nikolov I would like to ask you one more question. You have only mentioned the effect of peripheral glucagon, but do you have any comment on brain glucagon?

Lefèbvre Yes, certainly there is some glucagon in the brain, mainly in some species like the rat and, furthermore, extra-pancreatic sources of glucagon have also been proven to exist in the fundus of the stomach. Also in this connection, it has been claimed that there is glucagon in the salivary glands, but later it was shown that this was an artefact, because actually there was a compound destroying the tracer in the assay. Anyhow, I do believe that there is some glucagon in the brain, that the gene is probably there, and that some glucagon is produced there in minute amounts, although nobody knows what its effect can be. However, there are studies being done by colleagues in Japan which speculate about the possibility that glucagon may have an action on the regulation of appetite (In: Lefèbvre PJ ed. *Glucagon II. Handbook of Experimental Pharmacology. 66 II.* Berlin, Heidelberg, New York, Tokyo: Springer, 1983: 667–672).

Fehér My question is connected with the effect of glucagon on calcium metabolism. In our patient material there were two cases with a very severe tetany-like effect after using glucagon by infusion therapy. To counteract this effect we gave calcium to both of them and they recovered. In your opinion, do you think that this hypocalcaemia could be the result of the effect of glucagon on calcium metabolism?

Lefèbvre I have never studied that myself, so I do not have personal experience. However, I do know that it has been claimed that glucagon stimulates the release of calcitonin and that, of course, might explain the hypocalcaemia. I do not know to what extent this applies to man, but in *in vitro* systems, the calcitonin-releasing effect of glucagon is substantial.

Carr-Locke Can you tell me what the glucose load was that you gave in your exercise experiment?

Lefèbvre A hundred grams, although we did the same and got the same results when we gave four times 25 g.

Carr-Locke Why do you think there was an hour's delay in your exercise experiment between the start of exercise and the rise of glucagon?

Lefèbvre That is a very good question. The mechanism leading to the rise of glucagon in man during this type of exercise has been a matter of discussion; some believe that it is due to sympathetic activation, and I think that this is

13

because the sympathetic activation takes place slowly in that type of exercise. Therefore, this means that if we do more strenuous exercise glucagon will rise much more rapidly.

2
Effect of glucagon on haemodynamics and gastrointestinal tract motility. Role of the glucagon receptor

L. SANTAMARIA and E. DE MIGUEL

INTRODUCTION

Living organisms have the capacity to receive, internalize and transmit information which may be used in the process of some type of metabolic activity. In this connection, hormones play an important role in the regulation of metabolism. It is currently accepted that hormones are bearers of a message that they transmit to the 'target cells' which carry the specific receptors located in the plasma membranes of the cell; the signal that is generated from the binding of the hormone to its receptor will eventually affect an effector component.

It has long been known that glucagon exerts a vasoactive action on the hepatic[1] and other vascular beds[2], where very important vasodilating effects have been observed. On the basis of this evidence we may postulate the existence of glucagon receptors in some structure or structures that might have an outstanding role to play in hepatic haemodynamics and which it would be important to study and clarify. These receptors may be located on the cellular surface of the hepatocyte in connection with an adenylate cyclase complex[3], in a similar fashion to what is seen in other types of receptors located at many other sites[4,5], as for example the β-adrenergic ones.

By binding to its receptor, glucagon favours the activation of the catalytic

15

component. Adenylate cyclase activation increases the intracellular levels of cAMP or second messenger, which stimulates glucose production through glycogenolysis, neoglycogenesis and lipolysis.

The hormonal action of glucagon is regulated by a group of enzymes, phosphodiesterases, which degrade cAMP and by a protein from the regulating membrane called N, dependent on GTP.

It is currently accepted that the receptor and the regulating protein constitute an oligomeric form, independent from the enzyme, in which the receptor inhibits the interaction between N and GTP. The signal resulting from the binding of the hormone to its receptor antagonizes this inhibitory effect, which leads to an increased interaction between GTP and the N protein, and the conversion of the oligomeric form into a monomeric one, N protein-receptor, with the capacity to activate adenylate cyclase.

Cyclic AMP is an allosteric modulator of protein kinase which facilitates the dissociation of its two subunits and the catalytic component. Consequently, a phosphorylation of certain proteins takes place, such as those in microtubules, endoplasmic reticulum, etc.

Due to the capacity of glucagon to adapt to inert surfaces and to the low diffusion of iodized hormones towards the interior of tissue samples, it has not been possible to evaluate the results obtained in these experimental models.

Little is known about the mechanism of action of these receptors. Even though the vasodilating effects of glucagon are widely known, as has already been mentioned, this polypeptide appears to be less potent from a vasoactive point of view than other substances, such as histamine or prostaglandin E2, it has a slow onset of action, it is prolonged and is cumulative. Further to a hypothetical direct action mediated by specific receptors, it may also inhibit the vasoconstriction induced by noradrenaline[1]. Therefore, it would be highly interesting to establish functional and morphological relationships between a hypothetical glucagonergic receptor and the adrenergic receptor, since it is known that β-receptors play an important role in the hepatic vascular responses mediated by noradrenaline and adrenaline[1], which apart from their predominant vasoconstrictive effect may also act secondarily as vasodilators. Likewise, there is no doubt that both glucagonergic and adrenergic receptors would also take part in functions other than the haemodynamic ones in the hepatic blood flow, such as the regulation of glycaemia[6].

FUNCTIONAL ASPECTS OF GLUCAGONERGIC RECEPTORS

Glucagon is a polypeptide hormone with a great variety of actions apart from its well known hyperglycaemic action. When this hormone is injected in experimental animals at physiological doses, it usually produces a rise in the arterial flow to some organs, while at the same time it decreases vascular resistance[1]. However, at other locations it does not modify these parameters. The reason why this hormone has a haemodynamic action which differs according to the different parts of the body is not quite clear. This led us to study the location of glucagon receptors in different organs since we hypothesized that there could be a direct relationship between the number of glucagon receptors and sensitivity to the hormone.

In addition to the presence of glucagon receptors in the hepatocyte membrane[7-9], over the last years glucagoneric receptors have been identified in other cells, as for instance in the membrane of polymorphonuclear leucocytes, where they have been demonstrated by autoradiographic techniques that identify the binding of ^{125}I-glucagon[10]. Glucagon plays a role in the cellular metabolism of the liver determining ultrastructural modifications in the hepatocyte, as is the case of glucagon depletion and hyperplasia of the smooth reticulum observed by Striffler et al.[11]. The structural requirements of the glucagon molecule necessary for enabling a perfect interrelationship between it and its receptor have also been studied. In this connection, the persistence of the amino group and carboxy-terminal group of the molecule are highly significant[12].

Concerning the mode of action of glucagon, it is postulated that the binding of a specific receptor to an adenylate cyclase complex would mediate the various effects to the polypeptide[13]. Furthermore, the effects of certain glucagon fragments[14] obtained through enzymatic digestion of the polypeptide, such as the 1–21 fragment, have been studied, and it has been observed that this fragment also stimulates the adenylate cyclase complex, and that it is able to displace the native glucagon from the receptors of the cell membrane[15].

Physiologically, one of the best known aspects of the action of glucagon is that related to vascular tone and gastrointestinal tract motility, in other words, that covering the effects of the hormone on smooth muscle fibre.

The peptide acts as a vasodilating substance in the microcirculation, especially in the portal, mesenteric[2], and renal[16] beds. Surprisingly, the vasodilating effect demonstrated in the splanchnic vascular system is not as clear in the peripheral system as has been shown by some authors in the femoral bed of the dog[17].

Further to this action on vascular smooth muscle fibre the spasmolytic effect on the smooth muscle tissue of the digestive tract must also be considered[16]. Studies both in vitro and in vivo attempting to explain these actions have resulted in different theories. Thus it was speculated that the effect on muscle could be mediated by the release of catecholamines from the suprarenal medulla[18]; other authors demonstrated that glucagon decreased muscle tone in strips of duodenal muscle of the cat in vitro and that it inhibited contractions induced by the infusion of acetylcholine which led them to conclude that this hormone was able to show a certain direct antagonistic effect on cholinergic

17

receptors. However, other authors[19] refer to a preganglionic anticholinergic action on the intramural plexuses of the intestine rather than on the muscle cell receptors.

Nonetheless, it is also believed that the myorelaxant action of glucagon is direct and associated with the adenylate cyclase complex, since it has been proved that phosphodiesterase inhibitors such as papaverine and theophylline potentiate the glucagonergic effects[20]. In addition, glucagon activates the cyclic adenylic complex in several tissues and it may be concluded that intracellular cAMP modulates the action of the hormone, especially in the vascular system, and particularly in the renal artery, and that it may well regulate the calcium-dependent myorelaxant effect[21,22].

The spasmolytic effect of glucagon has been shown both in experimental animals and in man at different levels of the digestive tract such as the lower oesophageal sphincter, which it relaxes without affecting peristaltic waves[23,24], the stomach, gallbladder and small and large intestine[24].

If we accept that these actions of glucagon are receptor-dependent and consider that they vary according to the site of smooth muscle being studied[17,24], we may assume that a different distribution of the receptors exists at those sites, and therefore, there is a heterogenicity in the muscle tissue of the splanchnic and peripheral vascular beds and in the gastrointestinal tract from the point of view of the glucagonergic receptors. Thus, we tried to clarify the presence and distribution of these receptors, visualising them by means of autoradiographic techniques performed with ^{125}I-glucagon in several structures such as liver, small intestine, hepatic and renal arteries, portal vein and in arteries and veins of the femoral bed. Both in the case of the small intestine and the renal artery, ultrastructural autoradiographic studies have been performed[25–29], quantifying the silver grain distribution and evaluating the number of glucagon receptors[30,31].

LOCATION AND QUANTIFICATION OF RECEPTORS

In dog liver perfused with ^{125}I-glucagon, activity is made manifest in the form of grain tracks on the hepatocyte membrane, never in its nucleus and only occasionally on the cells of the sinusoidal lining (Figures 2.1 and 2.2). The track distribution spreads over the whole parenchyma with no special predilection for a certain site. They have also been observed on the portal space, on the walls of both veins and arteries (Figure 2.3). In sections taken from near the hilus hepatis, silver grains are also identified on the muscle fibres of the branches of the portal vein (Figure 2.4).

In the small intestine (jejunum) activity has been observed at the following sites:

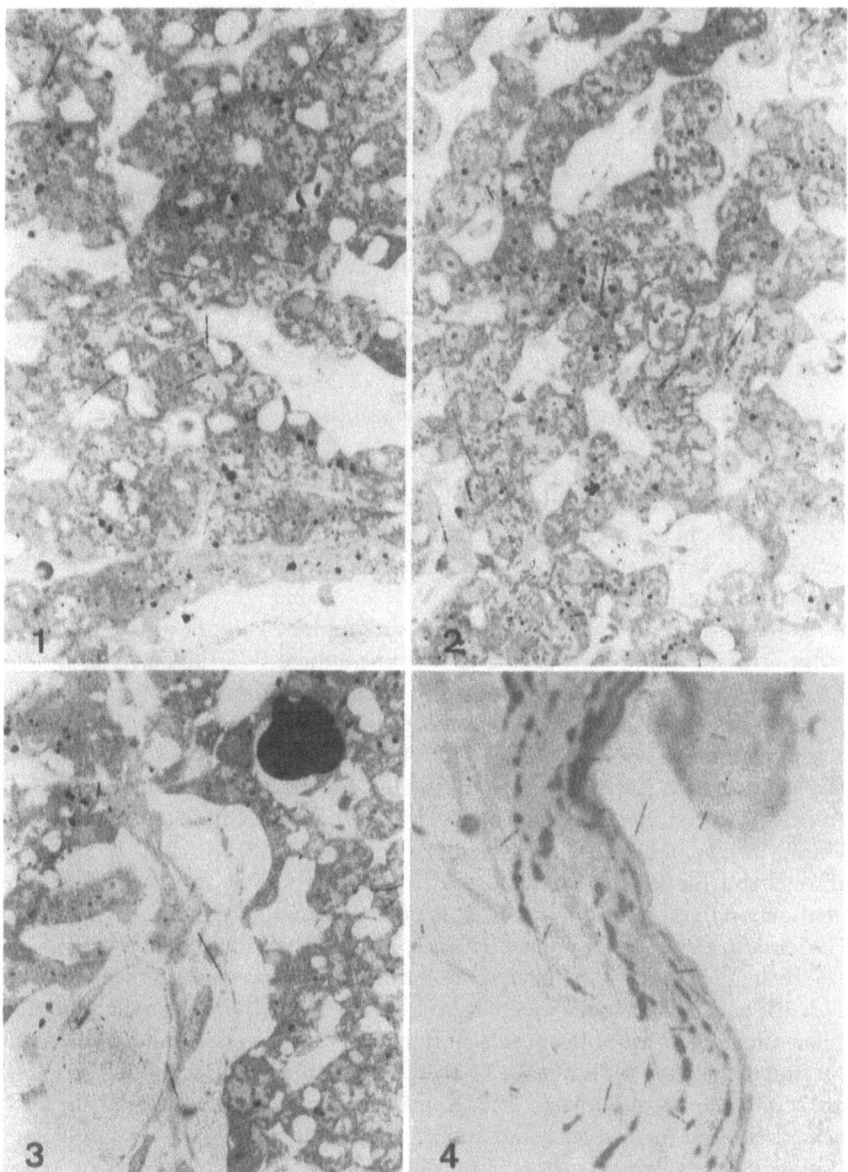

Figures 2.1 and 2.2 Detection of glucagon receptors on dog liver sections perfused with ^{125}I-glucagon and autoradiographed. Tracks are observed on the hepatocytes and occasionally on the sinusoid cells (× 400)

Figure 2.3 Detection of glucagon receptors. Tracks are observed in a portal space (× 400)

Figure 2.4 Detection of glucagon receptors. Tracks are found on the walls of the fibrous branches of the porta vein (× 400)

(1) First (in order of intensity of labelling) is the muscular layer, in which silver grains are seen near the membrane of the smooth muscle fibre (Figures 2.5 and 2.6). Labelling is also observed on the vascular muscle wall and occasionally in the pericytes of the arterioles and venules, but never in their endothelium.

(2) Second is the submucosa, where silver grains are also seen on the smooth muscle fibre or on the pericyte of arterioles and venules. The muscularis mucosae cells also show medium-intensity labelling.

(3) Third, quite unexpectedly, we found activity in the pericaryon of the ganglionic cells of the plexuses of Auerbach and Meissner (Figures 2.7 and 2.8).

(4) Finally, no significant labelling was observed in the lamina or epithelium of the cell.

In the femoral vascular bed (Figure 2.9) very scanty labelling of the arterial layer is seen. In the vein, tracks or isolated silver grains are observed in greater quantities than in the artery and are always located on the muscular structures of the vascular walls.

With ultrastructural quantitative autoradiography of the dog intestine, the silver grain distribution is such that it can be assumed that the activity of ^{125}I-glucagon bound to its receptor on the membrane of the smooth muscle cell is twice as much as the activity measured in the rest of the cellular and extracellular compartments studied (Figure 2.10).

The number of 'active sites' that can be related to the true number of receptors[29] located on the plasmalemma is 1582 ± 383 molecules μm^{-2}. In addition, the labelling seems to be highly specific since it is possible to identify a 60% shift of the labelled molecules if unlabelled glucagon is added to the incubation medium at a 3 $\mu mol\, l^{-1}$ concentration (Santamaría, L., De Miguel, E., Codesal, J., Ramírez, J. R. and Picazo, J., unpublished data).

The findings in the renal artery are similar to those described in the jejunum[30]. The distribution of activity of ^{125}I-glucagon is also twice as much in the plasmalemma of the smooth muscle fibre as it is in the remaining cellular and extracellular structures (Figure 2.11). In this case, the number of 'active sites' is 2607 ± 463 molecules μm^{-2}, 39% more than that of the intestinal smooth muscle cells. Also in this case the shift of the active molecule was significant (60%) when unlabelled glucagon (3 $\mu mol\, L^{-1}$) was added[31].

Further to the perfusion techniques with ^{125}I-glucagon, we also attempted the identification of glucagonergic receptors by means of direct incubation of unfixed tissue sections; however, this procedure is inadequate for several reasons: namely, damaging of the cells with cryostat, a higher background risk and lower resolution power of the method when compared to that of labelled

20

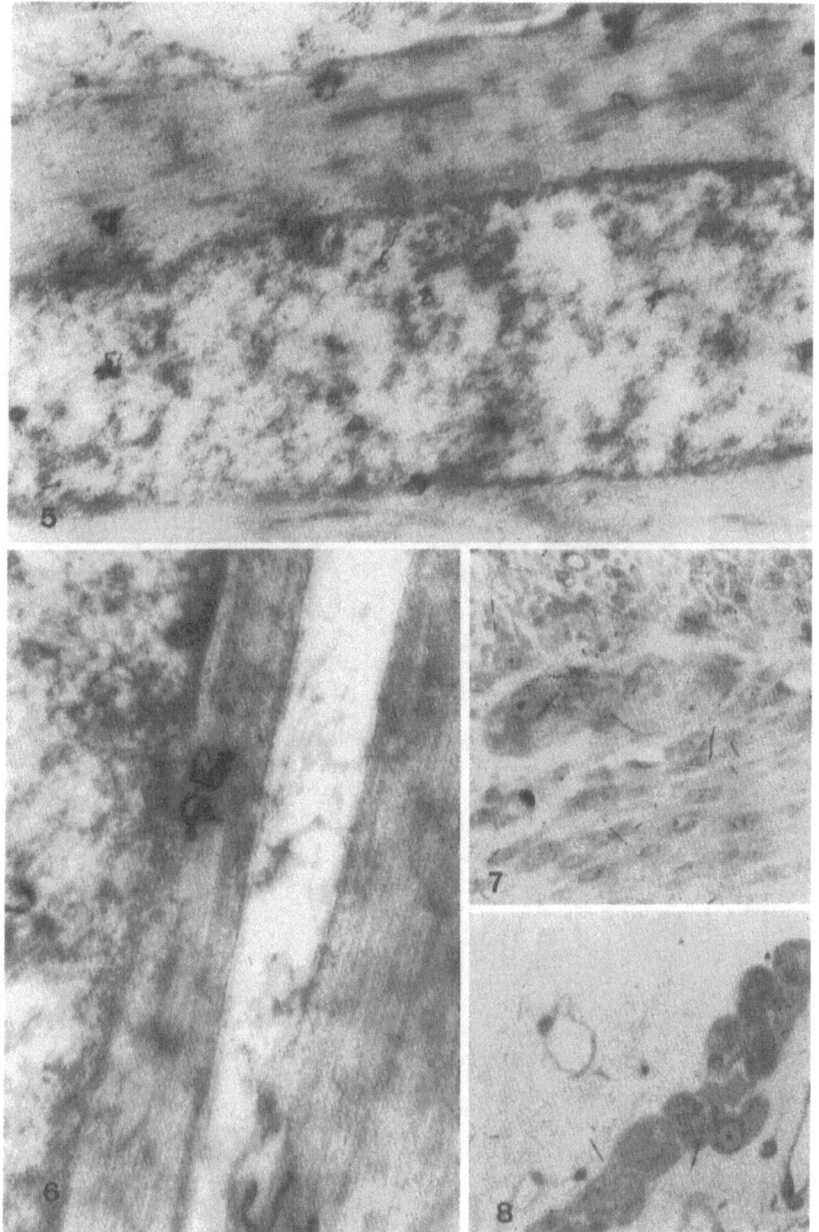

Figures 2.5 and 2.6 Electron radiography of the smooth muscle of the dog small intestine perfused with ^{125}I-glucagon and autoradiographed. Silver grains are observed in the proximity of the plasmalemma (× 15 000)

Figure 2.7 Neurons of the plexus of Meissner of dog small intestine perfused with ^{125}I-glucagon and autoradiographed. Tracks are observed on the pericaryon (× 400)

Figure 2.8 Neurons of the plexus of Auerbach of dog small intestine perfused with ^{125}I-glucagon and autoradiographed. Tracks are observed on the pericaryon (× 400)

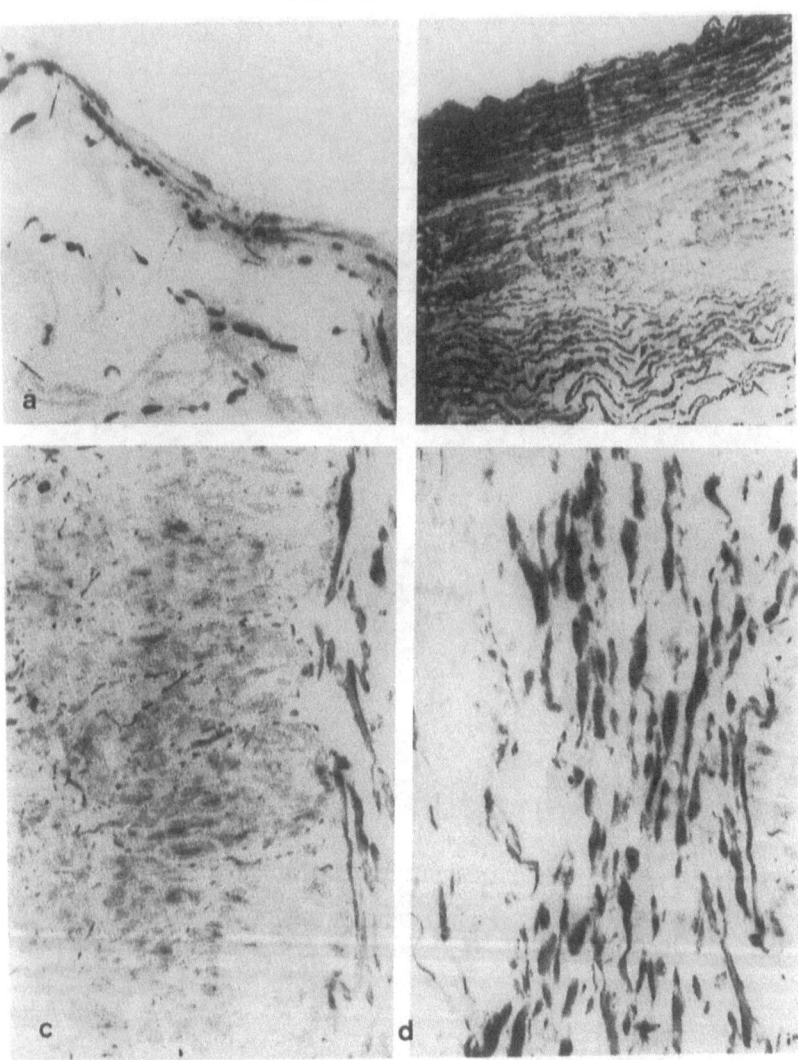

Figure 2.9 Perfusion of peripheral vessels with ^{125}I-glucagon. Autoradiographs of sections of: (a) femoral vein: activity in the form of tracks on smooth muscle fibres on the wall (× 400); (b), (c) and (d) femoral artery: absence of evident activity at all levels of the vascular wall (b: × 160; c: × 200; d: × 400)

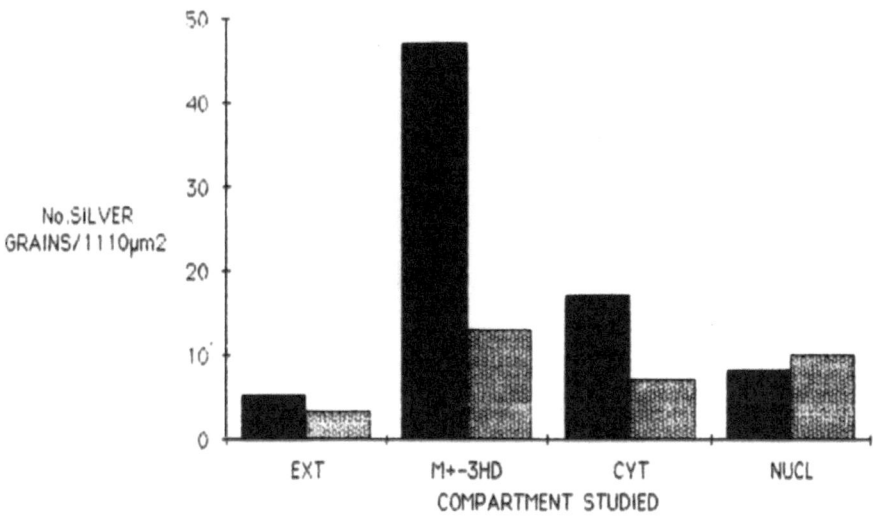

EFFECT OF GLUCAGON ON HAEMODYNAMICS

Figure 2.10
Plotting of silver grain distribution in the different cell compartments in dog smooth muscle
perfused with ^{125}I-glucagon and autoradiographed. EXT: extracellular; M$^+$-3MD: membrane;
CYT: cytoplasm; NUCL: nucleus. Black bars indicate perfusion with standard glucagon; dotted
bars control perfusion with labelled and unlabelled glucagon

glucagon perfusion. This is in agreement with Rogers[25] who stated that even
though the direct incubation technique can be of interest for the identification
of hormone receptors, it should be discarded for the same reasons that we
have mentioned.

The use of perfusion techniques with labelled hormones is the method of
choice for the visualization of their corresponding receptors[7,8], especially when
combined with fixation by aldehydes and inclusion in epoxy resins, since this
facilitates study by electron microscopy.

We would like to stress that in our study we have observed two different
silver grain distribution patterns on the emulsion deposited on the labelled
sections: as isolated grains and as short course tracks; these tracks always
appeared when we perfused ^{125}I-glucagon with a lower specific radioactivity.
This leads us to believe that in those instances the predominating factors of
the radioactive emission of the labelled material are very low energy electrons
present in the disintegration pattern of ^{125}I which by releasing that energy
very rapidly on very short courses through the emulsion generate the silver
grain tracks[25].

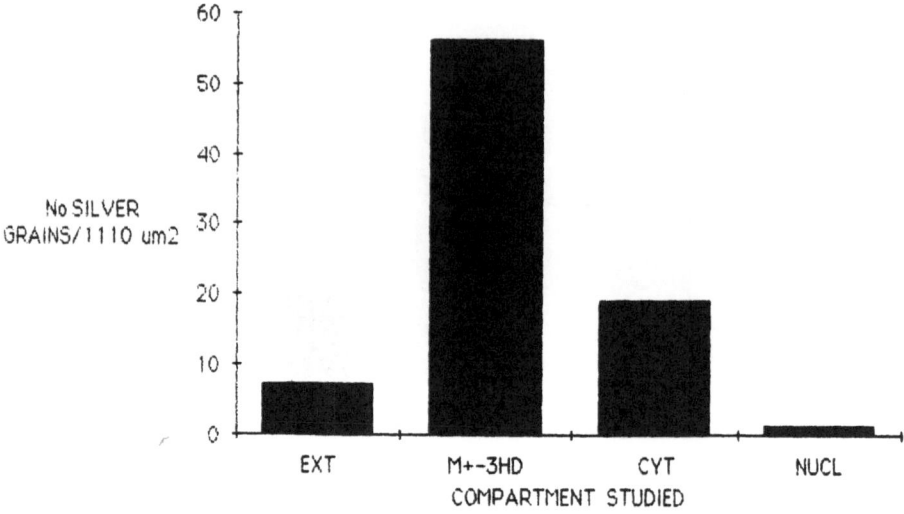

Figure 2.11 Plotting of silver grain distribution in the different cell compartments in dog renal artery smooth muscle perfused with ^{125}I-glucagon and autoradiographed. EXT: extracellular; M+-3MD: membrane; CYT: cytoplasm; NUCL: nucleus

DISCUSSION

From all this we can conclude that the presence of glucagon receptors in the hepatocyte membrane is confirmed by autoradiographic techniques, as has already been described by some authors[7,8].

Our findings in the small intestine are very interesting. We have been able to identify specific receptors for glucagon in the membrane of the smooth muscle fibre both on the intestinal wall and on the small and medium calibre vessels of the muscular and submucosal layers, but not in the lamina propria, which was to be expected since there is an almost total absence of smooth muscle cells in the vessels of the intestinal villi. We must also point out that no receptors were seen in the muscle of Brücke of the villi.

These findings are in agreement with the myorelaxant effect which, as seen earlier, has been described for glucagon both pharmacologically and physiologically[16,32]. In addition the results of the autoradiographic studies allow us to assume that, to a great extent, this myorelaxant effect is the result of a receptor-mediated direct action of glucagon on the smooth muscle fibre.

However, another highly significant finding worth mentioning is the presence of labelled sites in the neurons of the intestinal nervous plexuses since this suggests the possibility that glucagon may also act as a preganglionic blocker, as has already been pointed out in the past[16]. In fact the existence of hypothetical 'glucagonergic' nervous fibres which would release the hormone on the neuronal receptors just described, which would actually be located in postsynaptic structures of an inhibitory nature, appears as a strong possibility. Moreover, in the central nervous system there are nervous endings carrying peptides which behave immunohistochemically like glucagon, while in the intestine there are also nervous endings and neurons that secrete other vasoactive peptides such as VIP and Met-enkephalin[33]; however, up to date it has been impossible to identify neurons or neuroendings containing glucagon in the ganglions of the intramural plexuses of the intestine, in spite of different attempts to visualize them by immunocytochemical techniques.

In conclusion, we may say that there is a morphological and functional basis to believe that the spasmolytic effect of glucagon[19,32] can be mediated by the presence of specific receptors located primarily on the membrane of the smooth muscle cell (direct effect) and secondarily on the myenteric ganglia (indirect effect). The presence of receptors at this second location does not necessarily imply the existence of a synapsis which would have glucagon as the neurotransmitter.

Concerning the effect of glucagon on the vascular system, which has been widely studied in the past from a haemodynamic point of view[2,16], the autoradiographic technique has also demonstrated the presence of receptors in the smooth muscle cell of the different vascular walls studied. This is seen in the portal vein, both in the branches of the hilus hepatis or in the veins of the portal space as well as in the intestinal and renal vessels. The haemodynamic effects of glucagon on liver, intestine and kidney may be explained by the presence of these receptors, the activation of which would induce myorelaxation and therefore vasodilation with the consequent fall in blood pressure.

Receptors are also present in the hepatic sinusoidal endothelium, but in small amounts, and possibly this location has an exclusively metabolic effect, though it is also possible that here glucagon may act by inhibiting the hypothetical contractile mechanisms which would confer genuine sphincteric characteristics on certain parts of the endothelium of the sinusoid which would regulate blood flow through the liver[34-38].

Finally, it is also worth pointing out the almost total absence of receptors in the arteries of the femoral bed. This is in agreement with what has been described by Kazmers et al.[17] concerning the absence of a vasodilating response of the femoral bed of the dog to glucagon; however, the presence of receptors that we have shown on the venous part of this bed indicates that it may be possible to obtain a glucagonergic vasoactive response there.

Nonetheless, it is still not possible to say much about the intimate mechanism of action of glucagon on its receptor. There is no doubt that as with many other hormonal substances, the receptor may be bound to a second messenger system such as cAMP, but it remains to be known whether the myorelaxation seen after the activation of this system is related to the redistribution of the Ca^{++} ion as has been suggested by Andersson[21] and by Rasmussen[22], or whether the myorelaxant phenomenon depends on a more generalized metabolic action in which other glucagon-induced effects may play a role at an intracellular level, as would be the mobilization of the glycogen deposits of the smooth muscle cell or perhaps the inhibition of the effects mediated by other substances such as acetylcholine.

CONCLUSIONS

The present study leads to the conclusion that there are glucagonergic receptors in the liver which may have a haemodynamic role in addition to the metabolic one.

There are also glucagon receptors in the smooth muscle of the jejunum and renal vascular bed whose distribution confirms a direct role for glucagon in the motility and tone of the gastrointestinal and vascular smooth muscle fibre as well as its vasoactive role.

There is a heterogenicity between the splanchnic smooth muscle (vessels and walls of hollow organs) and the smooth muscle of the peripheral vessels (femoral bed) in the sense that at this latter location the role played by glucagon must be a limited one, judging from the scarce number of specific receptors.

The presence of glucagonergic receptors in the intramural neurons of the intestine leads us to suspect the possible existence of a preganglionic-blocking effect of glucagon which would inhibit intestinal motility. However, up to date it has been impossible to demonstrate the existence of glucagonergic neurons or nervous fibres by immunohistochemical techniques, so it is quite likely that the neuron receptors for glucagon may not be related to synapses where this hormone would act as a neurotransmitter.

References

1. Richardson PDI, Withrington PG. The vasodilator actions of isoprenaline, histamine, prostaglandin E2, glucagon and secretin on the hepatic arterial vascular bed of the dog. *Br J Pharmacol* 1976; 57: 581–588.
2. De Miguel E, Salgado G, Ginestal JM, Martínez-Veiga JL, Codoceo R, Santamaría L. Acción vasoactiva del glucagón sobre el sistema porta. I) Estudio en el sistema vascular mesentérico del perro. *Rev Esp Enferm Apar Dig* 1981; 59: 441–446.
3. Pohl SL. The glucagon receptor and its relationship to adenylate cyclase. *Fed Proc* 1977; 36: 2115–2118.
4. Lefkowitz RJ, Williams LT. Catecholamines binding to the β-adrenergic receptor. *Proc Natl Acad Sci USA* 1977; 74: 515–519.
5. Houslay MD, Ellory JC, Smith GA, Hesketh TR, Stein JM, Warren GB, Metcalfe JC. Exchange of partners in glucagon receptor-adenylate cyclase complexes, physical evidence for the independent, mobile receptor model. *Biochim Biophys Acta* 1977; 467: 208–219.
6. Forssmann WG, Ito S. Hepatocyte innervation in primates. *J Cell Biol* 1977; 74: 299–313.

7. Barazzone P, Gorden P, Carpentier JL, Orci L, Freychet P, Canivet B. Binding, internalization, and lysosomal association of ^{125}I-glucagon in isolated rat hepatocytes. A quantitative electron microscope autoradiographic study. *J Clin Invest* 1980; 66: 1081–1093.
8. Baumann G, Pnavilai G, Freinkel N, Domart AL, Metzger BE, Levene MB. Hepatic insulin and glucagon receptors in pregnancy: Their role in the enhanced catabolism during fasting. *Endocrinology* 1981; 108: 1979–1986.
9. Broer Y, Freychet P, Rosselin G. Insulin and glucagon receptor interaction in genetically obese Zucker rat. Studies of hormone binding and glucagon-stimulated cyclic AMP levels in isolated hepatocytes. *Endocrinology* 1977; 101: 236.
10. Bhathena S, Home S, Schoechter GP, Rodman RS, Wahl L, Recant L. Pequerie identification of human mononuclear leukocytes bearing receptors of somatostatin and glucagon. *Diabetes* 1981; 30: 127–131.
11. Striffler JA, Cardell EL, Cardell RR. Effects of glucagon on hepatic glycogen and smooth endoplasmic reticulum. *Am J Anat* 1981: 160: 363–379.
12. Bregman MD, Trivedi D, Hruby VS. Glucagon amino groups. Evaluation of modifications leading to antagonism and agonism. *J Biol Chem* 1980; 252: 11725–11731.
13. Epand RM, Rosselin G, Hui Bon Hoa D, Cote TE, Laburthe M. Structural requirements for glucagon receptor binding and activation of adenylate cyclase in liver study of chemically modified forms of the hormone, including N-trinitrophenyl glucagon, and antagonist. *J Biol Chem* 1981: 256: 1128–1132.
14. Hruby VS, Agarwal NS, Griffem A, Bregman M, Nugent CS, Brendel K. Glucagon structure-function relationship using isolated rat hepatocytes. *Biochim Biophys Acta* 1981; 674: 383–390.
15. Wright DE, Hruby VS, Rodbell M. A reassessment of structure-function relationships in glucagon. Glucagon 1–21 is a full agonist. *J Biol Chem* 1978; 253: 6338–6340.
16. Diamant B, Jørgensen KD, Weis JU. Structure-activity relationship for the spasmolytic action of glucagon. In: Picazo J, ed. *Glucagon in Gastroenterology and Hepatology*. Lancaster: MTP Press, 1982: 25–35.
17. Kazmers A, Whitehouse WM, Lindenauer SM, Stanley JC. Dissociation of glucagon's central and peripheral hemodynamic effects: Mechanism of reduction and redistribution of canine hindlimb blood flow. *J Surg Res* 1981; 30: 384–90.
18. Fasth S, Hultén L. The effect of glucagon on intestinal motility and blood flow. *Acta Physiol Scand* 1971; 83: 169–173.
19. Gagnon G, Regoli D, Rioux F. A new bioassay for glucagon, *Br J Pharmacol* 1978; 64: 99–108.
20. Bitar KN, Jensen RT, Gardner JD, Makhlouf GM. Secretin, glucagon and VIP receptors on isolated gastric smooth muscle cells: Physiological relevance. *Gastroenterology* 1982; 82: 1018.
21. Andersson RGG. Cyclic AMP and calcium ions in mechanical and metabolic responses of smooth muscles. Influence of some hormones and drugs. *Acta Physiol Scand* 1972; suppl 382: 1–59.
22. Rasmussen H. Ions and second messengers. In: Weissman G, Clayborne R, eds. *Cell Membranes Biochemistry, Cell Biology and Pathology*. Tucson: HP Books, 1976: 203.
23. Behar J, Field S, Marin C. Effect of glucagon, secretin and vasoactive intestinal polypeptide on the feline lower oesophageal spincter: Mechanism of action. *Gastroenterology* 1979; 77: 1001.
24. Hogan WJ, Dodds WJ, Hoke SE, Reid DP, Kalkhoff RK, Arndorfer RC. Effect of glucagon on oesophageal motor function. *Gastroenterology* 1975; 69: 160.
25. Rogers AW. *Techniques of Autoradiography*. 3rd edn. Amsterdam: Elsevier North Holland Biomedical Press, 1979.
26. Backett NM, Parry DM. A new method for analysing microscope autoradiographs using hypothetical grain distributions. *J Cell Biol* 1973; 57: 9–15.
27. Salpeter MM, Fertuck HC, Salpeter EE. Resolution in electron microscope autoradiography. III. Iodine-125. The effect of heavy metal staining and a reassessment of critical parameters. *J Cell Biol* 1977; 72: 161–173.

28. Salpeter MM, McHenry FA, Salpeter EE. Resolution in electron microscope autoradiography. IV. Application to analysis of autoradiographs. *J Cell Biol* 1978; 76: 127–145.
29. Fertuck HC, Salpeter MM. Quantitation of junctional and extra-junctional acetylcholine receptors by electron microscope autoradiography after ^{125}I-Bungarotoxine binding at mouse neuromuscular junctions. *J Cell Biol* 1976; 69: 144–158.
30. Santamaría L, De Miguel E. Localización de receptores para el glucagón en fibra muscular lisa intestinal y vascular en el perro. Utilización de técnicas autorradiográficas. *Rev Esp Enferm Apar Dig* 1985; 64: 301–308.
31. Santamaría L, De Miguel E, Codesal J. Detección de receptores para el glucagón en la arteria renal del perro. Determinación cuantitativa por medio de autoradiografía ultraestructural. *Cir Esp* 1986; 49: 1295–1301.
32. Miller RE, Chernish SM. The response of gastrointestinal tract motility to glucagon. In: Picazo J, ed. *Glucagon in Gastroenterology and Hepatology*. Lancaster: MTP Press, 1982; 37–53.
33. Kobayashi S, Suzuki M, Uchida T, Yanaihara N. Enkephalin neurons in the guinea pig duodenum: A light and electron microscopic immunocytochemical study using an antiserum to methionine. Enkephalin-Arg-Gly-Leu. *Biomed Res* 1984; 5: 489–506.
34. Greep RO, Weiss L. *Histology*. 3rd edn. New York: McGraw Hill, 1973.
35. Gelman S, Einst EA. Role of pH, pCO_2 and PO_2 content of portal blood in hepatic circulatory autoregulation. *Am J Physiol* 1977; 233: 225–262.
36. Swan KC, Reynolds DG. Adrenergic mechanisms in canine mesenteric circulation. *Am J Physiol* 1971; 17: 79–85.
37. Laine GA, Hall JT, Laine SM, Granger HJ. Trans-sinusoidal fluid dynamics in canine liver during venous hypertension. *Circ Res* 1979; 45: 317–323.
38. Aaron S, Fulton R, Mays ET. Selective ligation of the hepatic artery for trauma of the liver. *Surg Gynecol Obstet* 1975: 141: 187–189.

3
Glucagon in upper gastrointestinal radiology

M. MARUYAMA

INTRODUCTION

There have been a great number of reports on the effects of glucagon in gastrointestinal radiology[1-6], and as reported by Miller et al.[1,2], it is generally accepted that hypotonicity and hypomotility of the upper gastrointestinal (g.i.) tract can be more effectively induced by glucagon than by anticholinergics and that reduction of hydrochloric acid and peptic gastric secretion can also be achieved by glucagon.

In these reports, however, emphasis was placed on the favourable effects of glucagon while discussion of its comparison with anticholinergics was avoided because of the rather high incidence of side effects with anticholinergics and, furthermore, even less attention was paid to the improvement of the quality of radiology when visualizing subtle mucosal lesions.

In parallel, in Japan the diagnostic accuracy of g.i. radiology has been increased by the use of double-contrast techniques. The improvements in X-ray equipment and in the quality of contrast medium have greatly facilitated the establishment of double-contrast techniques, but the use of antifoaming agents, proteinolytic substances and anticholinergics as premedication is extremely important to attain diagnostic double-contrast imaging with optimal mucosal coating.

In Japan anticholinergics have been used widely for more than 20 years for the performance of double-contrast examinations, but their serious complications have rarely been reported. Recently, however, the increasing incidence of cardiovascular disorders in Japan has led to a transitional period of revision of the extended use of anticholinergics for this type of procedure.

In this paper, the current status of premedication for g.i. radiology in Japan is first introduced, the role of glucagon is then assessed in comparison with anticholinergics and, finally, our opinion on the optimal procedure for upper g.i. radiology is described.

GLUCAGON IN UPPER GASTROINTESTINAL RADIOLOGY IN JAPAN

The premedicating agents most commonly used in Japan for g.i. radiology are anticholinergics. Glucagon is not used routinely since the general attitude in Japan at present is that it is used only when anticholinergics are contraindicated. Generally accepted contraindications of anticholinergics are heart disease, glaucoma, prostate hypertrophy, paralytic ileus and hypersensitivity to anticholinergic agents (Table 3.1).

In our hospital, 68 408 g.i. radiologic examinations including 59 705 upper g.i. and 8703 barium enema examinations were performed between 1983 and 1986. Out of the 68 408 examinations, Coliopan (butropium bromide) was used in 24 501 (35.16%), Buscopan (hyoscine N-butylbromide) was used in 1825 examinations (2.7%), and glucagon was available in 192 of them (0.28%) (0.06% in upper g.i. examinations and 1.75% in barium enemas) as shown in Table 3.2. The age and sex distribution of patients receiving glucagon for upper g.i. examinations is shown in Table 3.3. It is of great interest that 88.6% (31/35) of the patients who received glucagon were over the age of 50 years. This figure clearly reveals that glucagon was used only in rather aged patients who had one or more contraindications of anticholinergic agents.

Hypotonicity and hypomotility of the upper gastrointestinal tract were successfully induced by the use of glucagon in all cases, but satisfactory mucosal coating was not obtained in the majority of them (Figure 3.1). Mucosal coating of barium for double-contrast imaging was better achieved by the use of anticholinergics (Figure 3.2) than by the use of glucagon (Figure 3.1). On the double-contrast image obtained with the use of glucagon (Figure 3.1), the so-called 'area gastricæ' was always faintly outlined, which might be due to the dilution of barium suspension owing to continuous gastric juice secretion.

There is no significant difference in the tonicity and motility of the stomach between the use of glucagon (Figure 3.1) and the use of anticholinergics (Figure 3.2).

Yamazaki et al.[7] reported that when glucagon was used as premedication for the double-contrast examination of the stomach, (1) barium coating was not as good as when using anticholinergics; (2) gastric juice secretion was not

Table 3.1   Contraindications of anticholinergics

1. Heart disease
2. Glaucoma
3. Prostate hypertrophy
4. Paralytic ileus
5. Hypersensitivity

Table 3.2   Gastrointestinal radiology: no. of examinations and use of Coliopan, Buscopan and glucagon (Cancer Institute Hospital, 1983–1986)

	No. of examinations
Total g.i. radiology	68 408
U.g.i.	59 705 (87.3%)
Barium enema	8 703 (12.7%)
Use of Coliopan	24 051 (35.25%)
Use of Buscopan	1 835 (2.7%)
Use of glucagon (u.g.i.)	38 (0.06%)
Use of glucagon (barium enema)	152 (1.75%)

Table 3.3   Age and sex distribution of patients who received glucagon in u.g.i. radiology (Cancer Institute Hospital, 1983–1986)

Sex	Age (years)					Total
	~49	50~	60~	70~	80~	
Male	2	7	4	9	2	24
Female	2	4	1	3	1	11
Total	4	11	5	12	3	35

inhibited; (3) barium flow into the duodenum was often observed due to relaxation of the pylorus.

COMPARISON BETWEEN GLUCAGON AND ANTICHOLINERGICS

As mentioned before, in our experience, hypotonicity and hypomotility of the upper gastrointestinal tract were successfully induced by the use of glucagon but no superiority of glucagon could be found compared to anticholinergics in the double-contrast examination of the stomach.

Hamabe et al.[8] also pointed out that there was not such a great difference in hypotonicity of the upper gastrointestinal tract and the occurrence of duodenal flow between glucagon and anticholinergics, but that barium coating

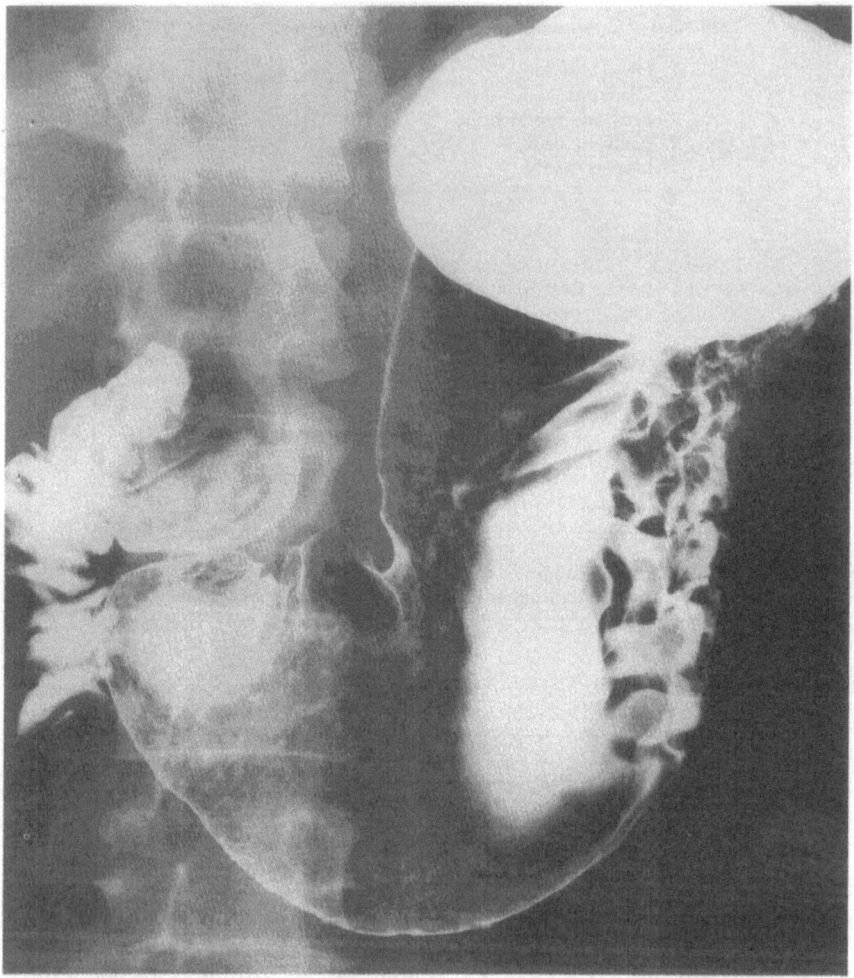

Figure 3.1 Double-contrast radiography taken with the use of glucagon (1 mg)

was obviously better when anticholinergics were used than when glucagon was used.

The main problem encountered when using anticholinergics as pre-medication to double-contrast procedures is their side effects. In the post-marketing surveillance of Coliopan (butropium bromide), its side effects were reported to have been observed in 1501 (12.43%) of 12 072 cases.

As characteristic side effects of anticholinergics (Table 3.4), thirst was

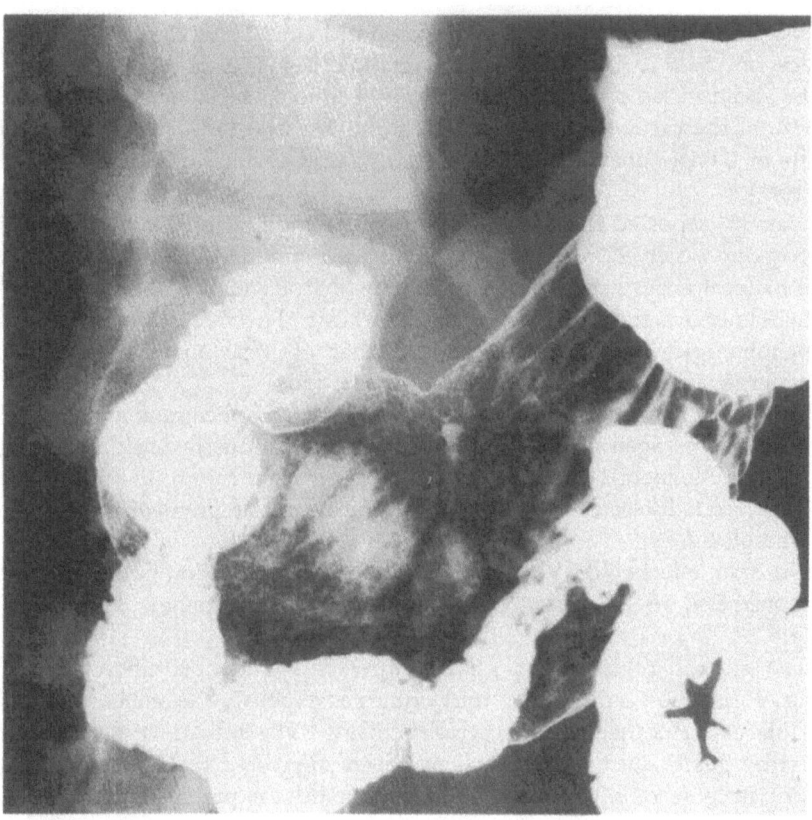

Figure 3.2 Double-contrast radiography taken with the use of an anticholinergic (Coliopan). A case of early cancer

Table 3.4 Side effects of Coliopan: no. of cases

Characteristic side effects		Prodromal symptoms of shock	
Thirst	917 (7.54%)	Facial flushing	65 (0.54%)
Palpitation	253 (2.10%)	Vertigo	32 (0.27%)
Sight disturbances	63 (0.52%)	Vomiting	22 (0.18%)
Dysuria	50 (0.41%)	Exanthema	12 (0.10%)
		Sweating	7 (0.06%)
		Chills	5 (0.02%)
		General flushing	1 (0.01%)
		Feeling of warmth	1 (0.01%)

encountered in 7.54% (911/12 072), palpitation in 2.10% (253/12 072), blurred vision in 0.52% (63/12 072), and dysuria in 0.41% (50/12 072).

In addition, as prodromal symptoms of shock, facial flush was noted in 0.54% of the cases, vertigo in 0.27%, vomiting in 0.18%, sweating in 0.06%, chills in 0.04%, general flushing in 0.02% and feeling of warmth in 0.01% (Table 3.4).

Namiki[9] reported that complications of premedication for gastrointestinal endoscopy occurred in 47 patients due to anticholinergics and in 43 patients due to local anaesthesia, including five deaths of which two were caused by anticholinergics and three by local anaesthesia. The rate of complications of anticholinergics is nearly the same as that of local anaesthesia, but anticholinergic agents are not prominently hazardous.

However, in view of the possibility of fatal complications and the recent increase in the aged population with contraindications to anticholinergics in Japan, anticholinergics should be used with extreme care in the future, which will undoubtedly lead to a wider use of glucagon as a premedication agent in g.i. radiology.

No toxic effects were encountered when using glucagon in our experience and, furthermore, the safety of glucagon has already gained general acceptance[1,2].

The greatest problem that glucagon presents is its cost efficacy. In Japan, 1 mg of glucagon is more than thirty times as expensive as an equivalent dose of Coliopan. Another problem which remains to be solved for glucagon is its effect on gastric juice secretion. It has been suggested that glucagon inhibits gastric juice secretion but, according to our own experience, glucagon does not seem to have an effect on that particular function.

PREMEDICATION FOR DIAGNOSTIC UPPER GASTROINTESTINAL RADIOLOGY

The double-contrast examination can be performed without premedication, but then mucosal coating is not satisfactory (Figure 3.3). The peristaltic wave has to be distinguished from a true deformity of the stomach. Therefore, in the radiologic diagnosis without premedication, both false negative and positive errors can occur.

In order to obtain the diagnostic double-contrast image of the stomach with a satisfactory mucosal coating, as already mentioned, not only is it necessary to achieve hypotonicity and hypomotility of the stomach in the first place but, additionally, gastric content should also be removed, and then gastric juice and acid secretion should be continuously inhibited.

The premedication sequence that we used to obtain optimal mucosal coating in the double-contrast examination of the stomach is shown in Table 3.5.

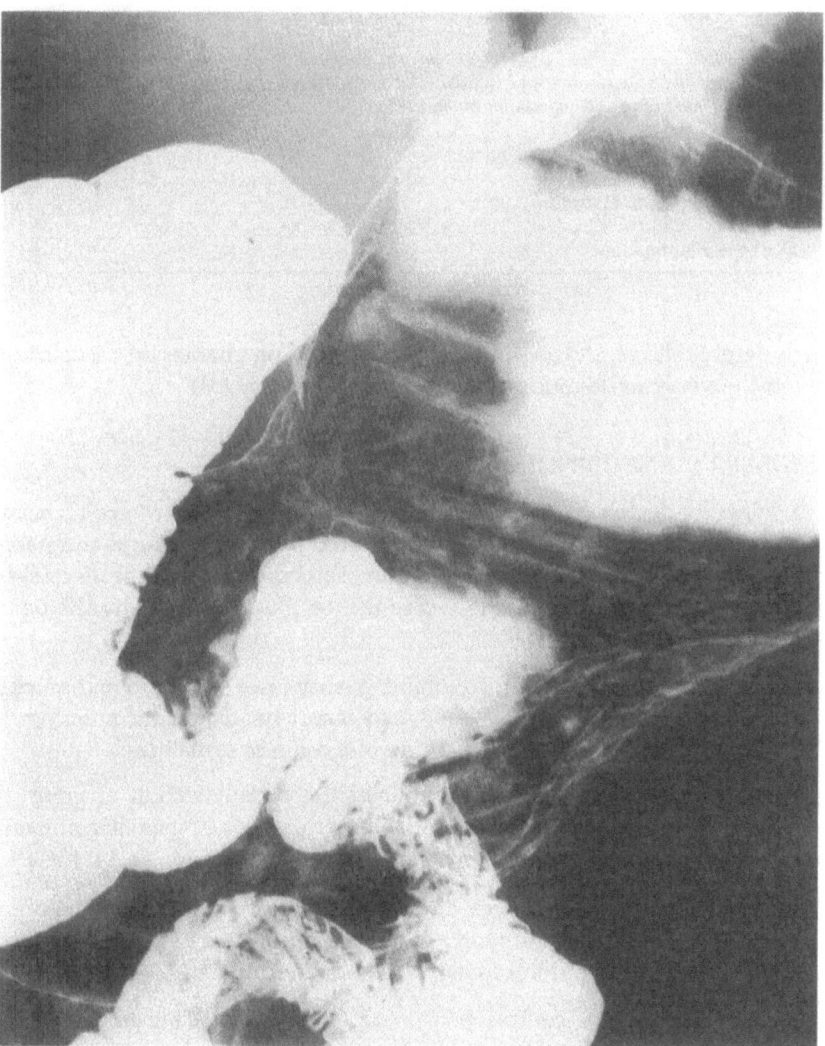

Figure 3.3 Double-contrast radiograph taken with the use of atropine sulphate and glucagon after oral administration of 250 ml of water containing pronase (2 g) and sodium bicarbonate (2 g)

Atropine sulphate 0.5 mg is injected intramuscularly and 250 ml of drinking water containing 2 g pronase and 2 g sodium bicarbonate is administered prior to examination. A nasogastric tube is inserted into the stomach to completely remove gastric juice and then 1 mg of glucagon is injected intramuscularly 10 min prior to the examination. With this premedication, the stomach is

Table 3.5 Sequence of premedication: method for obtaining optimal coating in detailed examinations

---

1. Two hours prior to examination: injection of atropine sulphate (0.5 mg), 250 ml of water including *pronase* (2 g) and *sodium bicarbonate* (2 g)

⇩

2. Intubation and removal of gastric juice

⇩

3. Injection of glucagon (1 mg)

⇩

4. Start of the examination

---

appropriately relaxed and an optimal mucosal coating enables the visualization of even the very subtle mucosal abnormalities (Figure 3.3).

SUMMARY AND CONCLUSIONS

(1) When performing diagnostic upper g.i. radiology, better results, including hypotonicity, hypomotility, inhibited hydrochloric acid and gastric juice secretion, and improved mucosal coating are not necessarily obtained more successfully by the use of glucagon than by the use of anticholinergics.

(2) Glucagon does not seem to inhibit gastric juice secretion and mucosal coating, which is the most important factor for diagnostic radiology, is not sufficiently good to detect fine mucosal abnormalities.

(3) Glucagon will play a leading role in the premedication of upper g.i. radiology, but it is very doubtful whether its use can yield benefit worth its cost, which is the main problem for the near future.

(4) Discussion should be directed not only to encouragement of the use of glucagon, but also to urgently solve the problems of cost and the poor effect on the inhibition of gastric juice secretion.

(5) Diagnostic double-contrast images capable of visualizing subtle mucosal lesions will be better obtained by the combined use of atropine sulphate, pronase, sodium bicarbonate and glucagon.

References

1. Miller RE, Chernish SM, Rosenak BD, Rodda BE. Hypotonic duodenography with glucagon. *Radiology* 1973; 108: 35–42.
2. Miller RE, Chernish SM, Skucas J, Rosenak BD, Rodda BE. Hypotonic roentgenography with glucagon. *Am J Roentgenol* 1974; 121: 264–274.
3. Meeroff JC, Jørgens J, Isenberg JI. The effect of glucagon on barium enema examination. *Radiology* 1975; 115: 5–7.

4. Kreel L. Pharmaco-radiology in barium examination with special reference to glucagon. *Br J Radiol* 1975; 48: 691–703.
5. Ishii H, Kamiya T, Oda Y, Okuno F, Takagi S, Aiso S, Yoshizawa M, Tsuchiya M. Hypotonic duodenography with the use of glucagon (Jap). *Nippon Shokakibyo Gakkai Zasshi* 1978; 75: 18.
6. Nomoto H, Kato T, Igarashi Y, Suzuki T, Watanabe H, Yokokura T, Sawano S, Nakazawa H, Iguchi S, Ishihara K, Mokonuma Y, Asahi R, Suzuki S. Application of glucagon to pharmaco-gastrointestinal radiology. Double blind trial (Jap). *Rinsho to Kenkyu* 1981; 58: 630.
7. Yamazaki H, Shimada T, Sukenaga T, Tanaka S, Takahashi H, Hayashi T, Miura T. Application of glucagon as a premedication drug in upper gastrointestinal X-ray examination (Jap). *Acta Med Chogo* 1984; 9: 53.
8. Hamabe S, Shinomura Y, Takahashi S, Kurokawa M, Himeno S, Saito R, Nonaka M, Tarui S, Ohnishi N, Hiraoka E. The use of glucagon for the upper gastrointestinal radiography in the aged. A double blind and crossover trial (Jap). *Nippon Shokakibyo Gakkai Zasshi* 1981; 78: 1585.
9. Namiki M. Complication at gastroenterological endoscopy (Jap). *Gastroenterol Endosc* 1984; 26: 2439.

DISCUSSION

Lefèbvre   Professor Maruyama, I think that you were very clear in showing the minor side effects of glucagon, but I think that there is one which should not be forgotten: If the patient has a known or unknown phaeochromocytoma, there can be a marked hypertensive crisis, because as you know from the literature, there have been three cases of phaeochromocytoma diagnosed on the occasion of such type of radiology using glucagon (Biggs I. *Br J Radiol* 1978; 51:981; Geelhoed GW. *Surgery* 1980; 87:719; McLoughlin MJ, Langer B, Wilson DR. *Radiology* 1981; 140:841). Did you see any of these three cases yourself?

Maruyama   No, I have not. We have documented several cases of phaeo-chromocytoma in our hospital, but those cases had already been diagnosed as such before using glucagon.

Lefèbvre   I would also like to comment in a different line, that I think the cost of glucagon is much too high for a compound which is very much used. Does anybody know whether there are plans to produce glucagon by genetic engineering,.which might reduce the price, or if it is already available by that method as has been done with insulin, growth hormone and other peptides? Because there was a time, about 15 years ago, when the cardiologists started to use huge doses of glucagon, 40–50 mg per day, and at that time there was a concern that they might use most of the existing glucagon and that then it would not be available for those in serious need of a glucagon shot to recover from hypoglycaemic coma.

Vilardell   Of course, as any other peptide, glucagon can be produced by genetic engineering and I can tell you that in fact work is now in progress for the production of glucagon by this method.

Nikolov   Dr Maruyama, could you explain with more detail your rationale for combining atropine with glucagon?

Maruyama   I selected atropine sulphate as the anticholinergic because this drug has less side effects than other anticholinergics such as hyoscine butyl-bromide or butropium bromide, and in order to inhibit the gastric juice secretion first. But atropine sulphate does not decrease motility, at least not as much as we expect. Therefore, we inject atropine sulphate first, 30 min to 1 h before starting the examination, so that gastric juice secretion is inhibited, and then, immediately before the examination we give glucagon to decrease or inhibit motility. It is by this procedure that we are able to obtain such beautiful mucosal details in the double-contrast examination. This is the reason why we use atropine sulphate first, with the purpose of inhibiting gastric juice secretion, and then, just before the examination glucagon, in order to inhibit motility itself.

Lefèbvre   I would like to add to Professor Maruyama's comment that the inhibition of gastric acid secretion is not due to glucagon but is probably more related to the glucagon-related compound oxyntomodulin, which has been identified and described by Bataille together with Victor Mutt (Bataille D, Coudray AM, Carqvist M *et al. FEBS Lett* 1982; 146:79–85).

Maruyama   Yes, I have read that publication, but it is just my impression, I do not have any evidence, that in X-ray examinations of the stomach the barium coating of the mucosal membrane is not as good when we use glucagon alone, and this may be explained by the fact that the gastric juice secretion is not actually inhibited by glucagon.

Nikolov   Professor Maruyama, in your patients, did you use 1 mg glucagon?

Maruyama   Yes.

Nikolov   However, there have been reports in the literature indicating that a glucagon dose as low as 0.1 mg provides adequate hypotonicity of the stomach, duodenum and small bowel for the biphasic gastrointestinal exam-ination (Miller RE, Chernish SM, Greenman GF, *et al. Radiology* 1982; 143: 317–320).

Maruyama   Yes, I understand your point, but in our practice and in Japan in general our doses in pharmacoradiology range between 0.5 and 1 mg of glucagon.

Baker   I am asking you this question as a non-radiologist and non-endoscopist and it goes back to what you said about the complications. Could you tell us a little bit more about the nature of the deaths that you saw with the local anaesthetic and the anticholinergics? That would seem to be a strong argument in favour of glucagon if you could get it to work as well as anticholinergics.

Maruyama   I have just seen one case of death during examination. I am very reluctant to say what kind of anticholinergic was used. This patient had a cardiac infarction requiring hospitalization one year before. He came to the hospital where I work and a resident injected the anticholinergic and started the examination. After giving one mouthful of barium in order to take the mucosal picture in prone position, our resident asked the patient to stop breathing, and just as he stopped breathing his heart stopped also. This is the only experience that I have had. I do not know the details of the other death and how it happened. This is my only experience.

4
Lower gastrointestinal tract radiology with glucagon

J. SKUCAS

INTRODUCTION

Although currently pharmacological agents are widely accepted throughout radiology, some radiologists still do not use these agents at all while others use them only for specific indications. In general, the advent of double contrast techniques and use of hypotonic agents has led to better colon relaxation and, hopefully, to a better diagnosis. With a double contrast barium enema there has also been less dependence upon post-evacuation radiographs.

A number of the early hypotonic agents were first adapted for use in the upper gastrointestinal tract. Some of these included morphine[1], propantheline bromide (Pro-banthine)[2-5], and atropine. Many of the earlier agents had undesirable side effects that at times were life-threatening[6].

While studying the effect of glucagon upon the gallbladder it was found fortuitously that duodenal hypotonia was produced following glucagon injection[7]. A subsequent study showed the value of glucagon as a hypotonic agent in hypotonic duodenography[8]. A follow-up double-blind, crossover study of the upper gastrointestinal tract showed that the hypotonic effect was better with glucagon than with propantheline or atropine[9]. An efficacy study of glucagon in the large bowel subsequently showed that the number and intensity of side effects encountered with glucagon was less ɯan with atropine[10]. Overall, the side effects with glucagon are minimal; one study found that the side effects of glucagon are similar to those with placebo[11]. In general, the patient is more comfortable, the large bowel is more dilated, fewer areas of spasm are encountered, and the overall interpretation of a barium enema appears to be easier. Without spasm, the examination can often be completed faster.

In adults, 1–2 mg of glucagon given intramuscularly leads to colon hypotonia beginning several minutes after injection and lasting for approximately 15 min. 0.5 mg of glucagon given intravenously has essentially the same hypotonic effect on the colon except that the onset is almost immediate and the hypotonia wears off approximately 10–15 min later[12]. Because of the cost of glucagon, most radiologists prefer the lower intravenous dose. Glucagon is not effective orally. In infants and children a dose of 0.8–1.25 $\mu g\,kg^{-1}$ intravenously has been found effective[13].

In the early 1970s it was proposed that hypotonia would help in the performance of a barium enema in the following conditions[14]:

(1) when the patient has painful spasm (Figure 4.1);

(2) when localized spasm is encountered, leading to confusion between spasm and benign or malignant strictures (Figure 4.2);

(3) for adequate distension during double-contrast studies;

(4) when there is functional inability to retain the enema;

(5) diverticular disease where spasm is encountered.

In 1980, Miller proposed that a double-contrast barium enema be performed for the following conditions[15].

(1) rectal bleeding;

(2) history of polyps or the detection of polyps on prior endoscopy;

(3) family history of neoplasms;

(4) patients over the age of 40 years;

(5) change in bowel habits, weight loss, unexplained anaemia, long-standing inflammatory disease, or other findings suspicious for colon cancer.

Many radiologists routinely use glucagon when performing a double-contrast barium enema. It is my impression that there is less use of glucagon in a private outpatient setting than in a hospital.

Several reports have described various sensitivity reactions associated with barium studies. Some of these reactions have occurred after a double-contrast barium enema *without* use of a hypotonic agent[16]. In one of these patients with urticaria, a skin prick test implicated methylparaben, a preservative used in the barium suspension, although the results were not fully conclusive. Sensitivity reactions have also been reported following the administration of barium suspension *and* the injection of glucagon[17]. In general, the incriminating agent

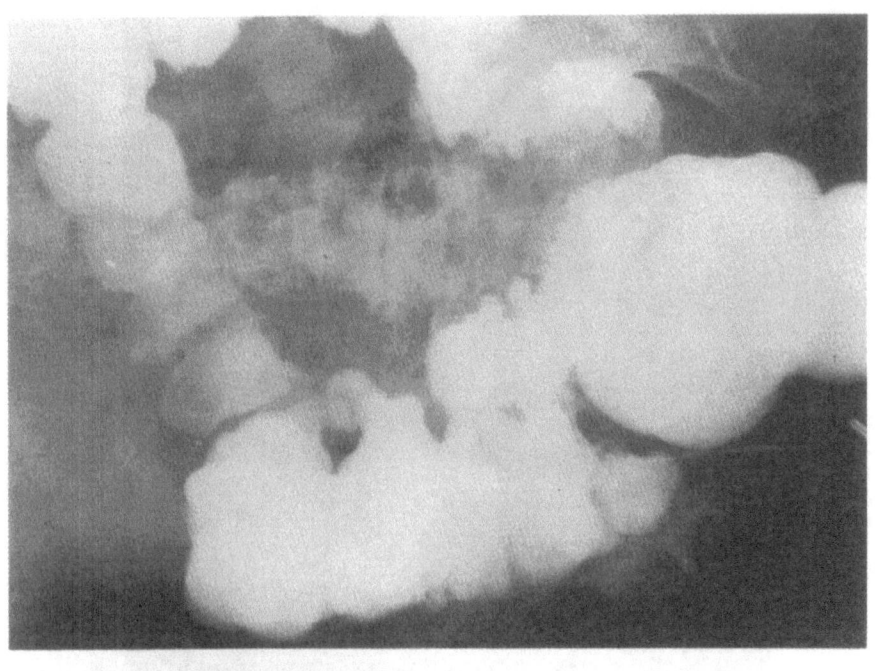

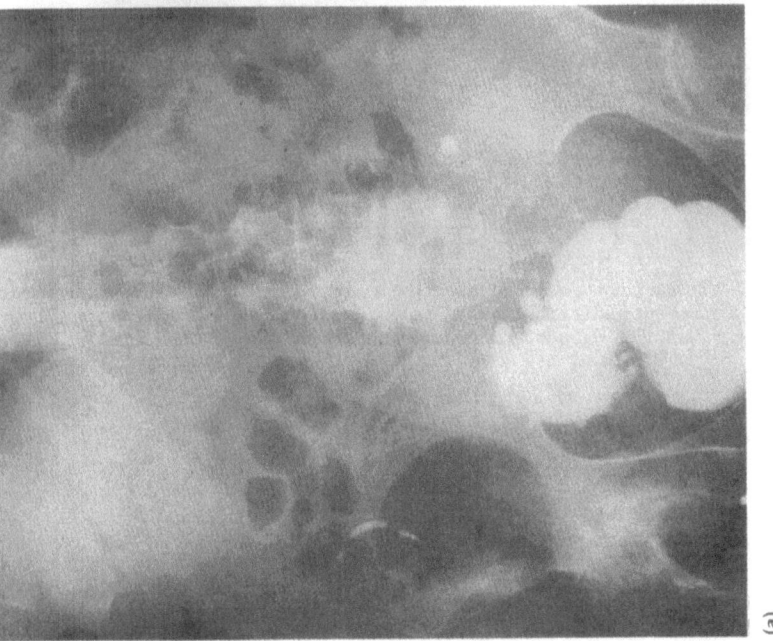

(b)

(a)

Figure 4.1 (a) An initial attempt at a barium enema was not successful because of spasm. Glucagon was not administered. (b) Following glucagon there is less spasm and the entire colon is filled.

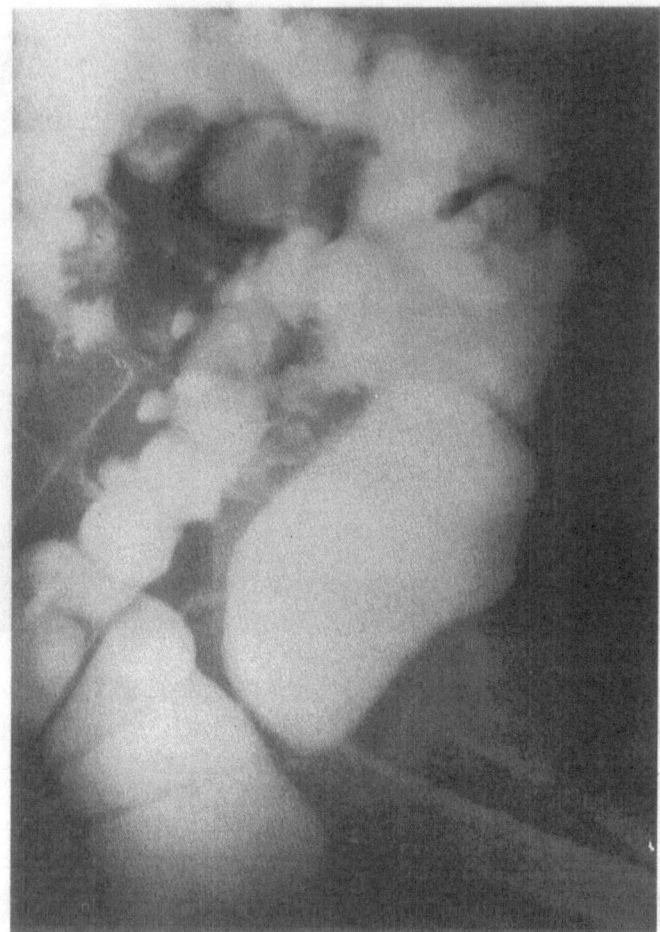

Figure 4.1 (c) A lateral view reveals contrast in the bladder. The patient had diverticulitis with a colo-vesical fistula. (From R.E. Miller and J. Skucas, *The Radiological Examination of the Colon*, Martinus Nijhoff Publ., The Hague, 1983, with permission)

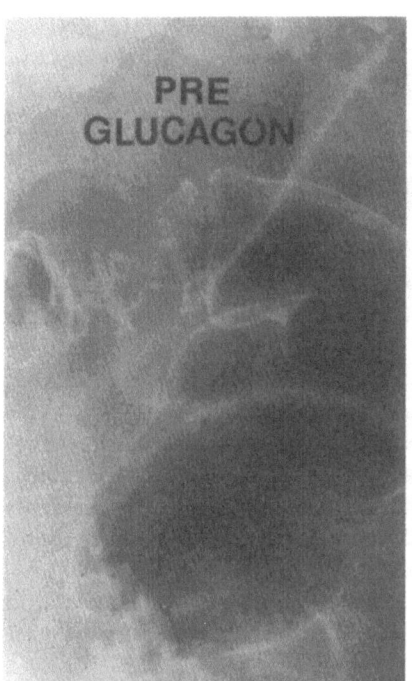
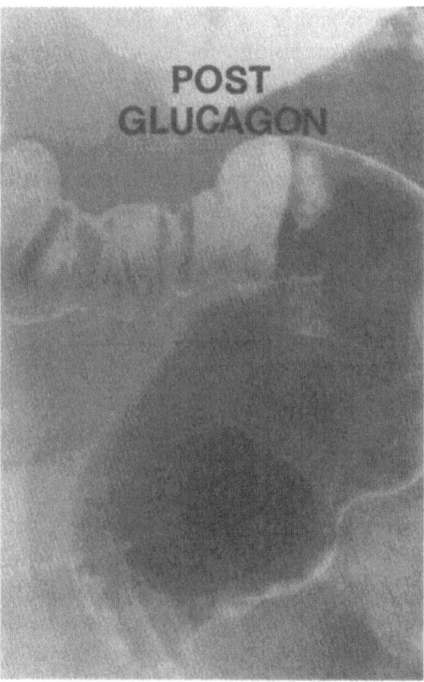

Figure 4.2 A narrowed segment was present in the sigmoid. To identify whether this segment was infiltrated by tumour or whether the narrowing is secondary to spasm, glucagon was administered. The sigmoid distended adequately; the previous narrowing was thus secondary to spasm. (From R.E. Miller and J. Skucas, *The Radiological Examination of the Colon*, Martinus Nijhoff Publ., The Hague, 1983, with permission)

has not been sought nor detected. Glucagon, however, has been incriminated in some reactions[18, 19], ranging from skin rash, periorbital oedema and erythema multiforme, to respiratory distress and hypotension. These reactions must be differentiated from the elevation in blood pressure found in patients with a phaeochromocytoma and the hypoglycaemia associated with an insulinoma[11, 20-23].

ACCURACY OF DIAGNOSIS

A number of studies have summarized the relative accuracy of a single-contrast *versus* a double-contrast barium enema. In general, these studies have concentrated on specific disorders, such as the detection of inflammatory bowel disease or the detection of polyps and cancers. Many of these studies were summarized by Miller and Skucas in 1983[24]. Over the years, nevertheless, the issue of single- *versus* double-contrast barium enema has been hotly debated, often at an emotional level. A number of recent studies have shown that the single-contrast barium enema is a sensitive examination in the detection of colon neoplasms[25-27]. The majority of studies have concluded, however, that the double-contrast barium enema is more accurate in detecting the extent and incidence of inflammatory bowel disease and in detecting colonic polyps[24, 28, 29]. The technique of examination is different between the two studies and many of the previous reports may be biased. The accuracy of each technique in the best of hands is difficult to gauge. One recent study comparing the relative accuracy of single-contrast *versus* double-contrast barium enema in the detection of colonic polyps found that the double-contrast barium enema was more effective in detecting polyps under 1 cm in size[30]. Both techniques detected 94–96% of polyps larger than 1 cm. In these patients 0.5 mg of glucagon was given intravenously. Yet even in this study an indirect bias exists; all of the studies were performed with remote control equipment and decubitus radiographs were not obtained. It is my opinion, shared by numerous residents over the years, that the two decubitus radiographs are the two most useful radiographs in a double-contrast barium enema.

Some investigators perform a single-contrast study in elderly and debilitated patients[30]. A double-contrast study can, however, be performed in the vast majority of patients over the age of 60[31].

Whether glucagon has been used in the examination or not has generally been relegated to secondary importance, at times not even being mentioned in a report. Although glucagon can make a barium enema examination more comfortable, few studies have looked at whether the use of glucagon indeed results in a more accurate diagnosis. Superficially at least, a more comfortable patient leads to a more relaxed patient with the radiologist thus being not as rushed to complete the examination. This question was addressed in one prospective, double-blind, crossover study[32]. Only patients with colonoscopic results were included. 133 patients were studied and each patient received either 1 ml of saline or 1 mg of glucagon in a double-blind fashion. Following completion of the double-contrast barium enema, a second injection of either glucagon or saline was given and the patient rotated 360°. Subsequently, four additional radiographs were obtained. These four radiographs, together with four corresponding radiographs after the first injection, were coded and interpreted in a blind manner by two radiologists. The degree of hypotonicity and quality of examination after glucagon were not significantly different from that seen after placebo. Although the sensitivity and specificity after glucagon were greater, the results were not statistically significant. These authors recommend that glucagon be used only in patients who exhibit significant discomfort during the examination, patients with diffuse or localized spasm, patients who have difficulty retaining the barium, and in patients with suspected colitis or diverticulitis[32]. These conclusions have been questioned because of the statistical methodology used[33], but the original conclusion still appeared valid in an extension of the study to 120 patients in each group[34].

The effect on patient comfort of substituting carbon dioxide (CO_2) in place of air during double-contrast examinations has been studied[35]. Patients in both groups received 1 mg glucagon intravenously. Out of 151 patients randomly assigned to the air or CO_2 groups, 30% of patients insufflated with air had 'relevant' pain, while only 11% of the CO_2 insufflated patients had similar pain. Likewise, post-evacuation radiographs revealed less residual gas in the CO_2 group. Several CO_2 delivery systems have been described[36, 37].

RETROGRADE ILEOGRAPHY

Some of the early investigators found that glucagon facilitated a retrograde small bowel examination[10]. This finding was confirmed by Violon et al. in 1981[38], who compared 52 patients who had not received glucagon with 50 patients who did receive glucagon during a double-contrast barium enema. In their 52 patients without glucagon, 15 showed barium filling of the ileum. In the 50 patients with glucagon, 37 had filling of the ileum. In addition, in the glucagon patients the terminal ileum tended to be outlined by double contrast, a finding rarely seen in the control patients. The finding that glucagon promotes reflux into the terminal ileum has been confirmed by other investigators[39]. When suspecting disorders involving the terminal ileum, such as Crohn's disease, some investigators have advised the routine use of glucagon[40]. Likewise, the treatment of meconium ileus and ileal plugs is believed to be aided by the use of glucagon[40].

COLONIC SPASM

The use of glucagon decreases the extent and severity of spasm encountered during a barium enema[10, 41, 42] (Figure 4.3). However, glucagon-resistant spasm is occasionally encountered in most practices. It has been my empiric observation that diabetic patients tend to have a higher incidence of glucagon-resistant spasm, although no formal study has been performed. Several investigators have had success in these patients by refilling the colon with a conventional single-contrast barium suspension[43, 44].

REDUCTION OF INTUSSUSCEPTION

Because of its ability to relax the bowel and promote ileal reflux, glucagon theoretically at least might have some value in reducing a colo-colic or an ileo-colic intussusception[40]. Fisher and Germann[45] reported two patients with

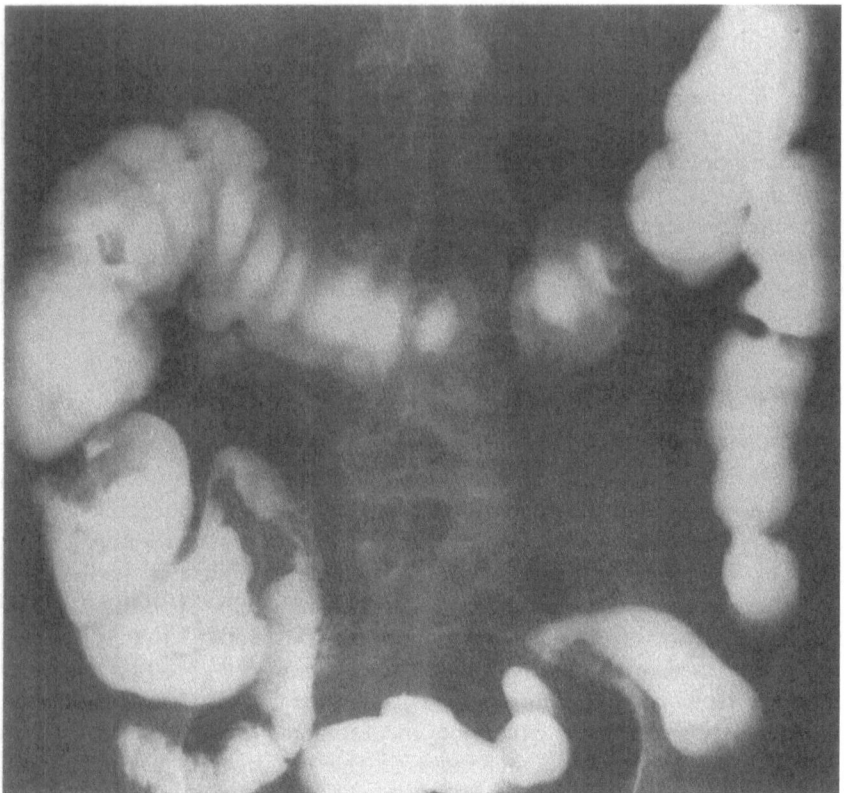

Figure 4.3 Two narrowed segments were found during a single-contrast barium enema. Glucagon had not been administered. Because the narrowing persisted, the radiologist concluded that two synchronous cancers were present. The patient underwent a laparotomy where no cancer was found. A subsequent double-contrast barium enema was normal

intussusception which could not be reduced with hydrostatic pressure alone but was reduced following the use of glucagon. Similarly, Hoy *et al.*[46] reported an 84% success rate in reducing intussusceptions when both glucagon and hydrostatic pressure was used. Occasional case reports of successful reduction of an intussusception credited glucagon for the success[47, 48]. One limited study showed that the success rate in reducing an idiopathic intussusception with the aid of glucagon is similar to that when hydrostatic pressure alone is used[40]. A subsequent, controlled, double-blind study in children gave a similar success rate for hydrostatic reduction with and without glucagon[49]. In this later study glucagon made no difference in the ease of reduction or the length of time needed for the reduction. A dose of $0.05\,\mathrm{mg\,kg^{-1}}$ (to a maximum of $1\,\mathrm{mg}$) intravenously was used. Some authors have given glucagon after a first failed hydrostatic attempt at reduction; the precise role of glucagon in this situation is difficult to gauge because simply by repeating hydrostatic pressure a second, third or even more times, improves the rate of successful reduction. A Scandinavian group encountered 69 patients with ileo-colic intussusception and gave them randomly 0.05 mg (kg body weight)$^{-1}$ of glucagon, intramuscularly, before start of the reduction[50]. In the groups with and without glucagon the rate of successful reduction was not statistically significant and the time for successful reduction, likewise, was similar. The patients in the control group who had three unsuccessful attempts at hydrostatic reduction then received glucagon and the fourth attempt at reduction was successful in 59% of the patients[50]. These investigators therefore concluded that there may be some benefit in using glucagon; their recommendation is that after two unsuccessful hydrostatic attempts at reduction of the intussusception, glucagon be administered before the next attempt is made[50].

PERORAL PNEUMOCOLON

When other examinations fail, the peroral pneumocolon examination is useful in evaluating the terminal ileum. Because of the increased incidence of ileo-colic reflux after the administration of glucagon[38], some investigators recommend routine use of glucagon for the pneumocolon examination[51].

COMPUTED TOMOGRAPHY

Computed tomography (CT) has been used as an aid in staging colo-rectal cancers. In particular, the presence of distal metastases and local extension outside the colon may be gauged by CT and aid the surgeon or therapist in designing an optimal approach. One study found that rectal distension with air, induced bowel hypotonia with glucagon (1 mg, intravenously), and intravenous opacification by contrast was helpful in evaluating the depth of tumour invasion[52]. The authors cautioned that full bowel distension is necessary to outline tumour extension. Glucagon was useful in preventing spasm and in achieving adequate distension.

Glucagon is often administered to patients undergoing abdominal CT examinations with an older scanner, where the scanning time is prolonged. The consequent decrease in peristalsis results in less motion artefacts. With the current fast scanners there is less need for bowel hypotonia. If glucagon is needed, a portable syringe pump to infuse glucagon can be used[53].

References

1. Porcher P. La stase duodénale provoquée. Procédé simple, rapide et fidèle, d'améliorer la visibilité radiologique et les détails de l'image du bulbe ulcéreux. *Arch Mal Appar Dig* 1944; 33: 24–26.
2. Baum M, Howe CT. Hypotonic duodenography in the diagnosis of carcinoma of the pancreas and its further use when combined with percutaneous cholangiography and pancreatic scintiscanning. *Am J Surg* 1968; 115: 519–525.
3. Bilbao MR, Rösch J, Frische LH, Dotter CT. Hypotonic duodenography in the diagnosis of pancreatic disease. *Semin Roentgenol* 1968; 3: 280–287.
4. Goldstein HM, Zboralske FF. Tubeless hypotonic duodenography. *J Am Med Assoc* 1969; 210: 2086–2088.
5. Merlo RB, Stone M, Baugus P, Martin M. The use of Pro-Banthine to induce gastrointestinal hypotonia. *Radiology* 1978; 127: 61–62.
6. Gelfand DW, Moskowitz M. Massive gastric dilatation complicating hypotonic duodenography. *Radiology* 1970; 97: 637–639.
7. Chernish SM, Miller RE, Rosenak BD, Scholz NE. Effect of glucagon on size of visualized human gallbladder before and after a fat meal. *Gastroenterology* 1972; 62: 1218–1226.
8. Chernish SM, Miller RE, Rosenak BD, Scholz NE. Hypotonic duodenography with the use of glucagon. *Gastroenterology* 1972; 63: 392–398.
9. Miller RE, Chernish SM, Skucas J, Rosenak BD, Rodda BE. Hypotonic roentgenology with glucagon. *Am J Roentgenol* 1974; 121: 264–275.
10. Miller RE, Chernish SM, Skucas J, Rosenak BD, Rodda BE. Hypotonic colon examination with glucagon. *Radiology* 1974; 113: 555–562.
11. Chernish SM, Davidson JA, Brunelle RL, Miller RE, Rosenak BD. Response of normal subjects to a single 2-milligram dose of glucagon administered intramuscularly. *Arch Int Pharmacodyn Ther* 1975; 218: 312–327.
12. Miller RE, Chernish SM, Brunelle RL. Gastrointestinal radiography with glucagon. *Gastrointest Radiol* 1979; 4: 1–10.
13. Ratcliffe JF. Glucagon in barium examinations in infants and children: special reference to dosage. *Br J Radiol* 1980; 53: 860–862.
14. Ferrucci JT Jr. Hypotonic barium enema examination. *Am J Roentgenol* 1972; 116: 304–308.
15. Miller RE. La radiologie du colon. *J Radiol* 1980; 61: 219–225.
16. Schwartz EE, Glick SN, Foggs MB, Silverstein GS. Hypersensitivity reactions after barium enema examination. *Am J Roengenol* 1984; 143: 103–104.
17. Gelfand DW, Sowers JC, DePonte KA, Sumner TE, Ott DJ. Anaphylactic and allergic reactions during double-contrast studies: Is glucagon or barium suspension the allergen? *Am J Roentgenol* 1985; 144: 405–406.
18. Harned RK, Stelling CB, Williams S, Wolf GL. Glucagon and barium enema examinations. a controlled clinical trial. *Am J Roentgenol* 1976; 126: 981–984.
19. Edell SL. Erythema multiforme secondary to intravenous glucagon. *Am J Radiol* 1980; 134: 385–386.
20. Lawrence AM. Glucagon. *Annu Rev Med* 1969; 20: 207–222.
21. Lawrence AM. Glucagon in medicine: new ideas for an old hormone. *Med Clin N Am* 1970; 54: 183–190.
22. Gomez-Pan A, Blesa Malpica G, Rodriguez Arnao MD, Oriol Bosch A. Glucagon as a drug. In: Picazo J, ed. *Glucagon in Gastroenterology.* Lancaster: MTP Press, 1979: 11–18.
23. McLoughlin MJ, Langer B, Wilson DR. Life-threatening reaction to glucagon in a patient with phaeochromocytoma. *Radiology* 1981; 140: 841–842.
24. Miller RE, Skucas J. *The Radiological Examination of the Colon.* The Hague: Martinus Nijhoff Publ., 1983.
25. Kaude JV, Harty RF. Sensitivity of single contrast barium enema with regard to colorectal disease as diagnosed by colonoscopy. *Eur J Radiol* 1982; 2: 290–292.
26. Teefey SA, Carlson HC. The fluoroscopic barium enema in colonic polyp detection. *Am J Radiol* 1983; 141: 1279–1281.
27. Johnson CD, Carlson HC, Taylor WF, Weiland LP. Barium enemas of carcinoma of the

colon: sensitivity of double- and single-contrast studies. *Am J Roentgenol* 1983; 140: 1143–1149.

28. Gelfand DW, Ott DJ. Single- *vs* double-contrast gastrointestinal studies: critical analysis of reported statistics. *Am J Roentgenol* 1981; 137: 523–528.
29. Winthrop JD, Balfe DM, Shackelford GD, McAlister WH, Rosenblum JL, Siegel MJ. Ulcerative and granulomatous colitis in children. *Radiology* 1985; 154: 657–660.
30. Ott DJ, Chen YM, Gelfand DW, Wu WC, Munitz HA. Single-contrast *vs* double-contrast barium enema in the detection of colonic polyps. *Am J Roentgenol* 1986; 146: 993–996.
31. Wolf EL, Frager D, Beneventano TC. Feasibility of double-contrast barium enema in the elderly. *Am J Roentgenol* 1985; 145: 47–48.
32. Thoeni RF, Vandeman F, Wall SD. Effect of glucagon on the diagnostic accuracy of double-contrast barium enema examinations. *Am J Roentgenol* 1984; 142: 111–114.
33. Marinelli D, Levine MS, Young M. Importance of sample size for statistical significance. *Am J Roentgenol* 1984; 143: 923–924.
34. Thoeni RFL. Importance of sample size for statistical significance (Reply). *Am J Roentgenol* 1984; 143: 924.
35. Coblentz CL, Frost RA, Molinaro V, Stevenson GW. Pain after barium enema: effect of CO_2 and air on double-contrast study. *Radiology* 1985; 157: 35–36.
36. Bessette JR, Maglinte DDT. Double-contrast barium enema study: simple conversion to CO_2. *Radiology* 1987; 162: 274–275.
37. Bernier P. Coblentz C. CO_2 delivery system for double-contrast barium enema examinations. *Radiology* 1986; 159: 264.
38. Violon D, Steppe R, Potvliege R. Improved retrograde ileography with glucagon. *Am J Roentgenol* 1981; 136: 833–839.
39. Monsein LH, Halpert RD, Harris ED, Feczko PJ. Retrograde ileography: value of glucagon. *Radiology* 1986; 161: 558–559.
40. Mandell GA, Teplick SK. Glucagon – Its application to childhood gastrointestinal radiology. *Gastrointest Radiol* 1982; 7: 7–13.
41. Gohel VK, Dalinka MK, Coren GS. Hypotonic examination of the colon with glucagon. *Radiology* 1975; 115: 1–4.
42. Meeroff JC, Jorgens J, Isenberg JI. The effect of glucagon on barium-enema examination. *Radiology* 1975; 115: 5–7.
43. Levine MS, Gasparaitis AE. Barium filling for glucagon-resistant spasm on double-contrast barium enema examinations. *Radiology* 1986; 160: 264–265.
44. Demas BE, Margulis AR. Combined use of double- and single-contrast barium enema in the evaluation of suspected colonic disease. *Gastrointest Radiol* 1984; 9: 241–245.
45. Fisher JK, Germann DR. Glucagon-aided reduction of intussusception. *Radiology* 1977; 122: 197–198.
46. Hoy GR, Dunbar D, Boles ET. The use of glucagon in the diagnosis and management of ileocolic intussusception. *J Pediatr Surg* 1977; 12: 939–944.
47. Lanocita M, Castiglioni G. Impiego del glucagone nella riduzione dell'invaginazione intestinale; presentazione di un caso. *Radiol Med* (Torino) 1980; 66: 513–516.
48. Coppola V, Verrengia D, Esposito F, Rossi R, Carbonara A. L'ausilio del glucagone nella riduzione idrostatica dell'invaginazione in corso di clisma opaco. *Minerva Pediatr* 1983; 35: 881–884.
49. Franken EA Jr, Smith WL, Chernish SM, Campbell JB, Fletcher BD, Goldman HS. The use of glucagon in hydrostatic reduction of intussusception: A double-blind study of 30 patients. *Radiology* 1983; 146: 687–689.
50. Mortensson W, Eklöf O, Laurin S. Hydrostatic reduction of childhood intussusception. *Acta Radiol Diagn* 1984; 25: 261–264.
51. Kelvin FM, Gedgaudas RK, Thompson WM, Rice RP. The peroral pneumocolon: its role in evaluating the terminal ileum. *Am J Roentgenol* 1982; 139: 115–121.
52. Hamlin DJ, Burgener FA, Sischy B. New technique to stage early rectal carcinoma by computed tomography. *Radiology* 1981; 141: 539–540.
53. Kreel L, Bydder G. Use of a portable syringe pump for glucagon administration in abdominal computed tomography. *Radiology* 1980; 136: 507–508.

DISCUSSION

Vilardell   I guess there is really no doubt that glucagon is very effective in colon radiology and, as a matter of fact, we use it quite often in our own institution for that purpose as well as for colonoscopy ...

Lefèbvre   Dr. Skucas, would you advise the use of glucagon 0.5 mg intravenously? Is that what you recommend?

Skucas   Yes; although some radiologists use 0.25 mg simply to save on the cost, primarily in a private patient setting, in many hospitals the usual dose is 0.5 mg.

Lefèbvre   I am saying this because from the metabolic point of view, even 0.5 mg is much too high a dose; as you know, you can get the same effects with 0.1 or even 0.05 mg ...

Skucas   Yes, of course, but radiologically speaking, I can say that we and others have found that different parts of the gastrointestinal tract respond differently to different doses. For example, in the stomach 0.1 mg intravenous is sufficient (Miller RE, Chernish SM, Greenman GF, *et al. Radiology* 1982; 143: 317–320). However, a similar dose in the colon is not sufficient to induce adequate hypotonia. In the colon one has to use a dose five to ten times as high as that for the stomach (Miller RE, Chernish SM, Brunelle RL. *Gastrointest Radiol* 1979; 4: 1–10). I think that that is where the variation comes in.

Maruyama   Have you encountered any patients in whom glucagon was not effective, I mean, in whom glucagon could not inhibit the motility of the colon?

Skucas   Yes; particularly I have found that in many diabetics it simply does not work. In general, when we still see spasm after using glucagon, the usual procedure is to give a second dose, but even then in many diabetics it does not work.

Lefèbvre   This problem that you have raised about the apparent lack of efficacy of glucagon in diabetics is extremely interesting and intriguing. From the metabolic point of view, diabetics usually have high circulating glucagon levels, and glucagon is extremely active in all metabolic parameters; with doses ten thousand times lower than those that we are talking about here, we are able to see increases in blood glucose levels, in free fatty acid levels, and in ketone bodies; so, from the metabolic point of view, diabetics are extremely and exquisitely sensitive to glucagon, and therefore it is hard to figure out why there is a lack of effect; but, of course, on the other hand, most diabetics have some degree of autonomic neuropathy, and the explanation may be that, in some way, this is responsible for the lack of effect of glucagon. Whether this has been published or documented I do not know, but I think that this lack, or relative lack of efficacy of glucagon in diabetics is an extremely important finding.

Skucas   As far as I know, this has not been published. Over the years, several of us have discussed this informally, but to my knowledge, nobody has set up a formal study of this particular phenomenon.

Carr-Locke   I have not observed this either, because I am not a radiologist, but my radiologists who use glucagon quite frequently for enemas and other procedures have never mentioned this to me.

Lefèbvre   But what about endoscopic procedures? Have you not been able to observe a lack of effect of glucagon in diabetics in this indication?

Carr-Locke   No, we have not specifically studied diabetics so, of course, I cannot really answer that, but I have never come across this phenomenon.

Lefèbvre   So I think maybe this is something we should think about in terms of setting up a formal study to evaluate the effect of glucagon in diabetics undergoing hypotonic radiology or endoscopic procedures.

Carr-Locke   I would like to add another question there. Might it be that, because diabetics have high circulating levels of glucagon, their receptor sites, wherever they are, are already occupied far greater than normal?

Lefèbvre   I do not think that this is the case, because all the metabolic effects are working perfectly, but still, I must admit that I am very surprised by this.

Vilardell   I think it would be important to know in the first place what kind of diabetics show that sort of response, because if you have, as Professor Lefèbvre said, diabetics who already have an advanced autonomic neuropathy with enlarged stomachs, which do not empty at all, and that type of dilated bowels, as you can see on X-ray, maybe glucagon alone will be unable to correct the disturbance which is already present. I wonder whether that is what is going on ...

Lefèbvre   Professor Vilardell, this is exactly what I have been trying to say and you have said it in better words. Usually these patients have gastroparesis and colonic paresis, and indeed, maybe it is simply because of that.

Skucas   It could very well be, but I do not know.

5
Glucagon in digestive endoscopy – its usefulness for premedication

T. TAKEMOTO, K. OKITA, M. TADA, H. KAWANO, T. YOSHIDA and T. AKIYAMA

INTRODUCTION

Anticholinergic agents have been used as premedication in digestive endos-copy, and their use is very convenient from a cost-benefit relationship point of view. However, the higher age groups population is increasing all over the world and, along with the older age, the medical treatment of those patients reaches a crucial point. In other words, elderly people often carry different kinds of complications which may hinder the gastrointestinal endoscopic examination. According to our experience, anticholinergic agents were not administered in 7.1% of a total of 10 574 patients examined by endoscopy between 1977 and 1986. On the other hand, when the age group older than 65 years was considered, it was evident that anticholinergics could not have been given to 19.5% of those patients because of contraindications such as glaucoma and prostatic hypertrophy, amongst others (Table 5.1).

Glucagon has been shown to have a relaxing effect on the tone and motility of the smooth muscle, when administered intravenously or intramuscularly for routine roentgen examination and endoscopy of the upper gastrointestinal tract[1-6], and also to be devoid of anticholinergic effects. Therefore, glucagon can be used as premedication for radiological and endoscopic procedures

Table 5.1 Cases in whom anticholinergic agents could not be used in our institution (Yamaguchi University, 1977–1986). Note that the cases unable to receive anticholinergic agents increased particularly among senile cases over 65 years

Total number of cases:	10 574	
anticholinergics were not administered in	753	(7.1%)
Number of cases over 65-years-old:	2 729	
anticholinergics were not administered in	531	(19.5%)

involving the gastrointestinal tract in elderly patients. We present here our experience with the pharmacological effects of glucagon on these structures.

GLUCAGON AS PREMEDICATION FOR UPPER GASTROINTESTINAL ENDOSCOPY

Several clinical studies have shown that glucagon can be used in endoscopy of the upper gastrointestinal tract[7–9], particularly when a 'quiet' field is necessary, e.g., for the removal of polyps or foreign bodies, or for the obtaining of biopsy samples or optimal pictures.

Our own study consisted of a group of 159 cases (84 males and 75 females) who were undergoing gastrointestinal endoscopy. Five minutes before starting the procedure, patients received 1 mg glucagon intramuscularly. After the injection, changes in gastric tone and motility were assessed according to Niwa's criteria (Table 5.2). In 140 of the 159 patients studied, peristalsis of the stomach was inhibited to such a degree that endoscopy could be performed without any obstacles (Table 5.3). The usefulness of glucagon as a premedicating agent was evaluated by several attending endoscopists. As shown in Table 5.4, in 81.8% of the cases glucagon was considered to be a useful premedication in this field.

In two of the 159 cases, increased salivation was reported as an adverse effect. Furthermore, a transient increase in blood sugar levels was observed in all 159 patients when this parameter was measured within one hour after glucagon administration (Figure 5.1).

These results allow us to confirm glucagon as a valuable adjunct in gastrointestinal endoscopy.

GLUCAGON AND INTRALUMINAL OESOPHAGOGASTRIC MANOMETRY

Inhibition of oesophageal and gastric motility with glucagon was studied using intraluminal oesophagogastric manometry. Pressures were measured following the method illustrated in Figure 5.2. After insertion of the catheter, a dose of 10 mg metoclopramide was given intramuscularly in order to enhance

Table 5.2 Criteria for judging gastric motility (modified Niwa's classification)

Grade	Criteria for judgement
I	No peristalsis
II	Slight peristaltic movement
III	Moderate peristaltic movement
IV	Strong peristaltic movement
V	Markedly increased peristaltic movement

Table 5.3 Effect of glucagon on gastric motility

| | Grade of gastric peristalsis | | | | Total |
I	II	III	IV	V	cases
70 (44.0%)	70 (44.0%)	13 (8.2%)	6 (3.8%)	0	159

Table 5.4 Usefulness of glucagon for premedication as judged by endoscopists

Good	69 (43.4%)
Fair	61 (38.4%)
Slightly disturbed	29 (18.2%)
Disturbed	0
Total cases	159

oesophageal and gastric peristalsis, this was followed by the administration of 1 mg glucagon. Pressures were continuously monitored according to the continuous station technique. It was observed that the administration of metoclopramide produced an increase in peristalsis of these organs, which was inhibited remarkably soon after the injection of glucagon. The case depicted in Figure 5.3 represents an example of the effect seen in this group. It is clearly shown that intra-oesophageal and gastric pressures, which increased after metoclopramide administration, were depressed abruptly within 1 min after glucagon injection.

SPHINCTER OF ODDI MOTILITY AND GLUCAGON

Endoscopic retrograde cholangiopancreatography (ERCP) is the most useful diagnostic imaging technique for the evaluation of diseases involving the biliary tract. Also, when performing ERCP, an adequate premedication is important as a means of improving the rate of successful cannulations of the papilla of Vater.

Motility and pressure of the duodenum and the sphincter of Oddi were

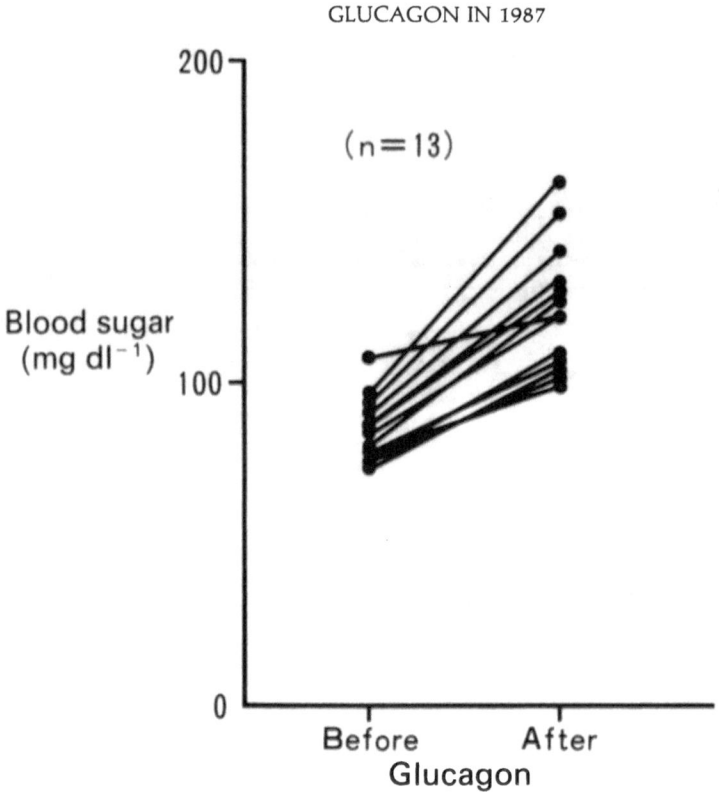

Figure 5.1 Changes in serum blood sugar one hour after injection of 1 mg glucagon

measured before and after the administration of glucagon in a group of four healthy individuals (three males and one female), who volunteered for a manometric study. Intraluminal pressures of the duodenum and the papilla of Vater were measured using a microtransducer (Miller Instruments Co., USA). As a first step, the duodenoscope was inserted into the second portion of the duodenum and the microtransducer was introduced through the biopsy channel and left in place for measurement of duodenal pressure. Thereafter, this microtransducer was positioned in the papilla of Vater to record pressures in this area.

In all four subjects pressures in both regions were reduced immediately after the administration of glucagon. As shown in Figure 5.4, after glucagon injection both duodenal maximum wave amplitude and mean pressure were reduced. As far as sphincter of Oddi motility is concerned, it was shown that the mean

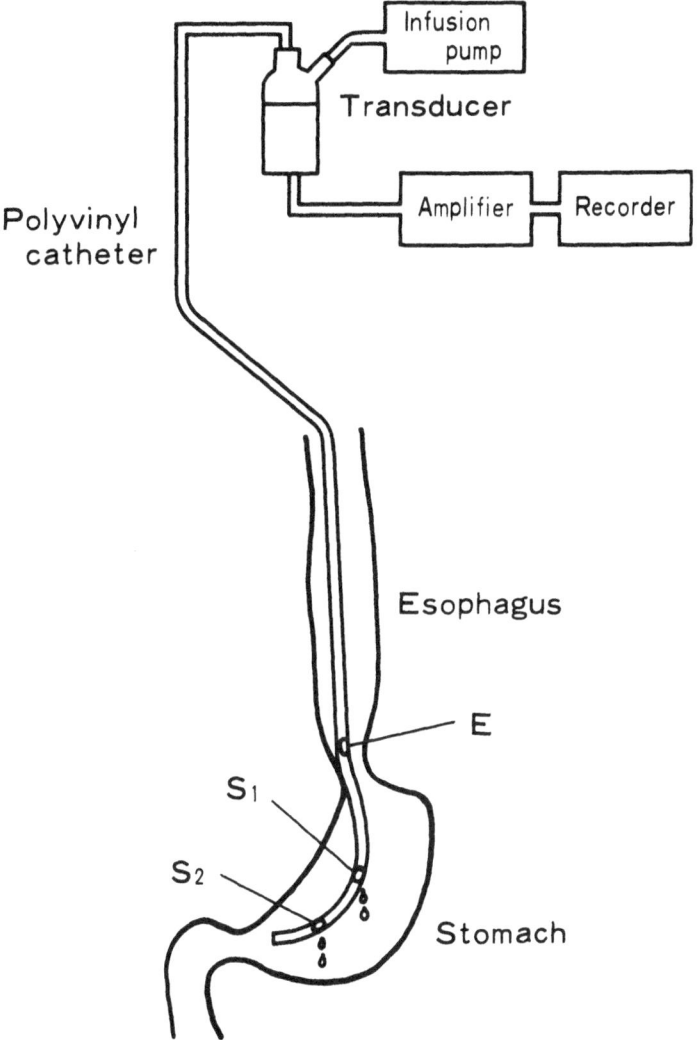

Figure 5.2 Measurement of intraluminal oesophagogastric pressure

systolic and diastolic pressures of the papilla of Vater decreased after the administration of glucagon (Figure 5.5).

In addition to changes in motility, the duration of the relaxing effect of glucagon was evaluated and compared with that of prifinium bromide. It was found that the duration of the effect of glucagon on duodenal and sphincter of Oddi motility was much longer than that of prifinium bromide.

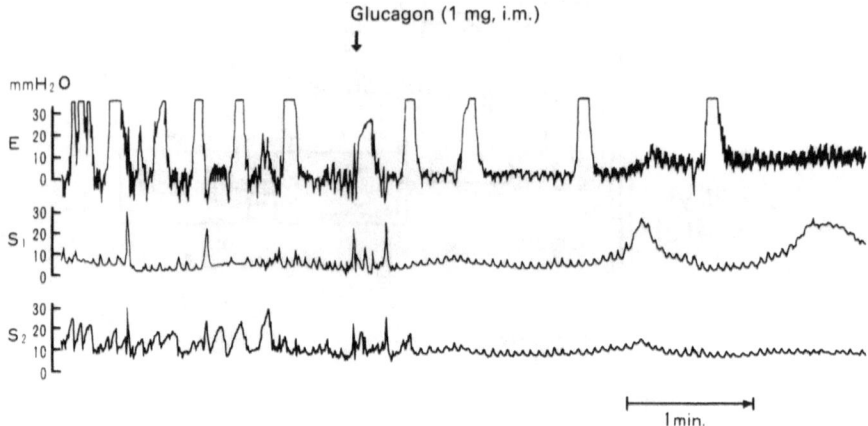

Figure 5.3 Changes in oesophagogastric manometry after glucagon administration. This result was taken from a healthy 21-year-old female volunteer

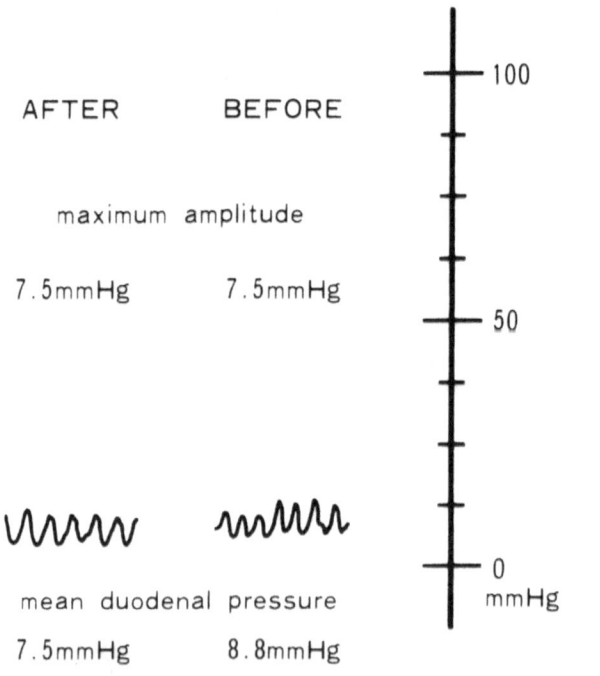

Figure 5.4 Changes in duodenal pressure before and after glucagon administration

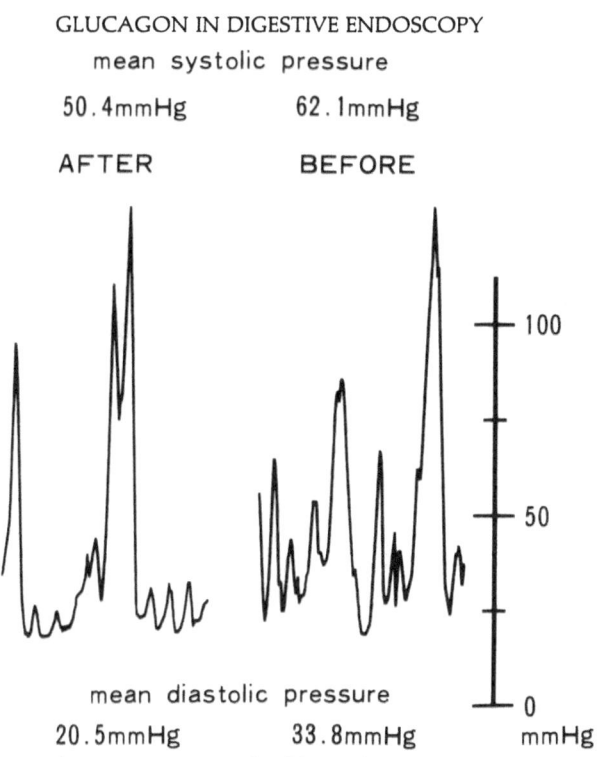

mean systolic pressure

50.4mmHg   62.1mmHg

AFTER   BEFORE

100

50

mean diastolic pressure

20.5mmHg   33.8mmHg   0

mmHg

Figure 5.5   Changes in spincter of Oddi motility after glucagon injection

These results confirm that glucagon is a useful premedication for ERCP.

COLONIC MOTILITYAND GLUCAGON

It has been reported that glucagon inhibits both slow wave electrical activity and motility throughout the colon by a direct effect on the colonic smooth muscle[10]. Chowdhury and Lorber[11,12] found that glucagon inhibited food- and morphine-induced motor activity of the distal colon and rectum, and significantly decreased the motility index of the hyperactive segment of the rectosigmoid junction[13].

We studied the effect of glucagon on neostigmine-stimulated colonic motility in five patients, using a colon fibrescope[14]. The method used was the following: the scope was inserted from the anus to the ascending colon, where the first open-tipped catheter filled with water was placed. Then the scope was drawn back to the transverse colon, where the second catheter was also left. The third catheter was left indwelling at the sigmoid colon through a sliding tube (Figure 5.6). After 30 min, basal colonic intraluminal pressure was recorded

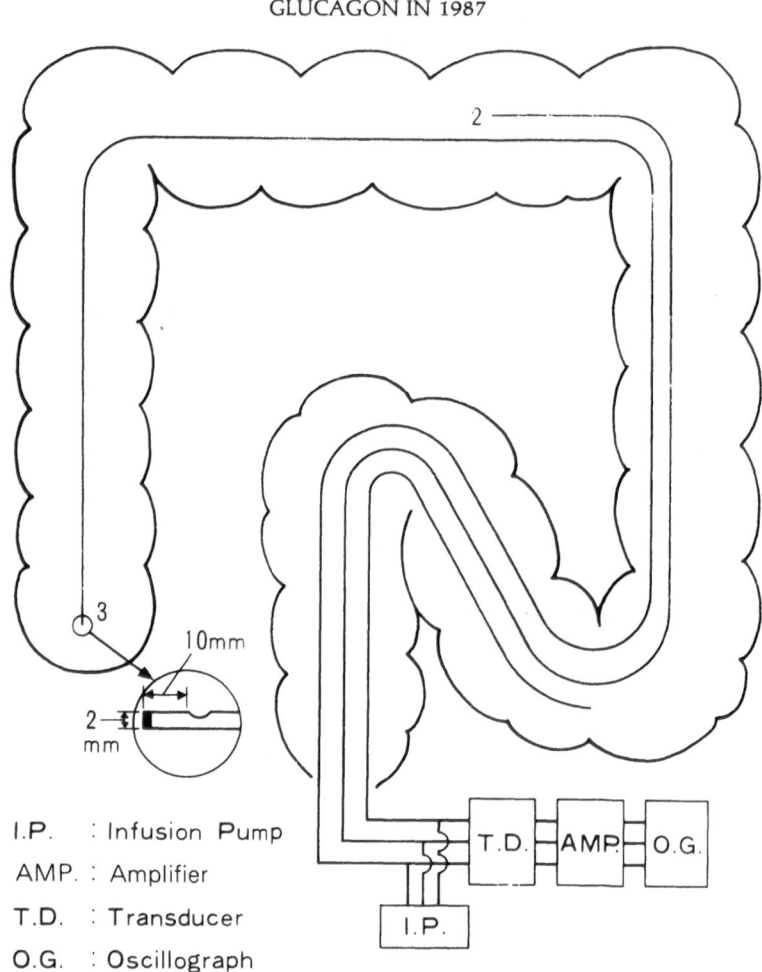

I.P.   : Infusion Pump
AMP. : Amplifier
T.D.   : Transducer
O.G.   : Oscillograph

Figure 5.6   Measurement of colonic motility

for 15 min. Subsequently 0.5 mg neostigmine was administered intramuscularly and colonic motility was recorded for an additional 30 min. Then 1 mg glucagon was injected and pressure recording was continued for another 15 min. As shown in Figure 5.7, an increase in colonic motility was elicited by the administration of neostigmine, and the subsequent injection of glucagon resulted in a remarkable inhibition of motility in all three colonic segments assessed. The average duration of the inhibitory effect of glucagon was 11 min. The motility pattern from one patient, which is illustrated in Figure 5.7, was similar in all five patients studied.

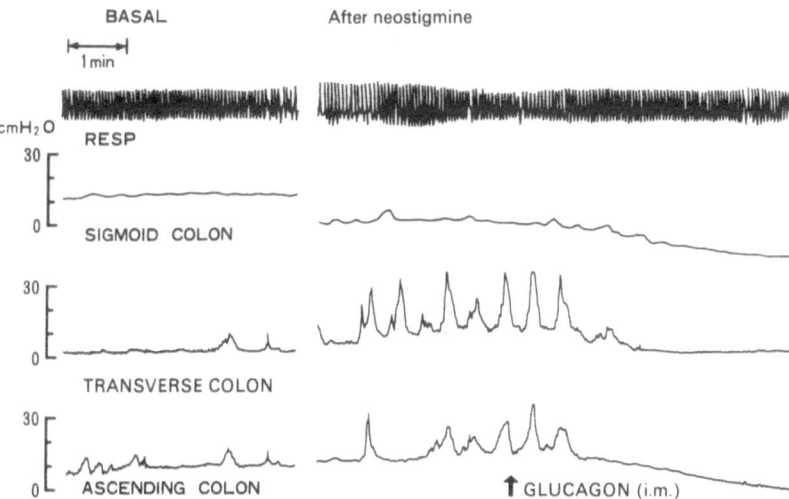

Figure 5.7 Changes in colonic motility measured at the sigmoid colon, transverse colon and ascending colon after treatment with neostigmine and glucagon. Note that glucagon remarkably inhibited neostigmine-induced increase in motility

These results support the usefulness of glucagon as premedication for colonoscopy and barium enema examination.

CONCLUSIONS

Glucagon has a strong inhibitory effect on the motility of the digestive tract and sphincter of Oddi, which make it the drug of choice for digestive endoscopy and radiographic barium enema examination of the colon. However, from the cost–benefit point of view, the use of glucagon as premedication in these procedures should be limited to aged patients with glaucoma, prostatic hypertrophy or other contraindications to the use of anticholinergics.

Acknowledgement

We are indebted to Drs Y. Okazaki, T. Fuji and T. Harima for their contribution to this study.

References

1. Chernish SM, Miller RE, Rosenak BD, Scholz NE. Hypotonic duodenography with the use of glucagon. *Gastroenterology* 1972; 63: 392–398.
2. Miller RE, Chernish SM, Skucas J, Rosenak BD, Rodda BE. Hypotonic roentgenology with glucagon. *Am J Roentgenol* 1974; 121: 264–274.

3. Bertrand G, Linscheer WG, Raheja KL, Woods RE. Double-blind evaluation of glucagon and propantheline bromide (Pro-Banthine) for hypotonic duodenography. *Am J Roentgenol* 1977; 128: 197–200.
4. Qvigstad T, Larsen S, Myren J. Comparison of glucagon, atropine, and placebo as premedication for endoscopy of the upper gastrointestinal tract. *Scand J Gastroenterol* 1979; 14: 231–235.
5. Kawamoto H *et al.* Effect of glucagon on the upper gastrointestinal motility. *Gastroenterol Endosc* 1983; 25: 1347.
6. Stoecker R, Foy D. Improvement of gastric mucosal detail in the double-contrast upper gastrointestinal examination utilizing low-dose glucagon. *J Am Osteopath Assoc* 1984; 83: 660–662.
7. Hradsky M, Stockbrügger R, Dotevall G, Ostberg H. The use of glucagon during upper gastrointestinal endoscopy. *Gastrointest Endosc* 1974; 20: 162.
8. Giesen HK. Kardiale Nebenwirkungen der Osophago-Gastro-Duodenoskopie in Abhängigkeit von der Prämedikation. *Dtsch Med Wsch* 1978; 103: 1517–1520.
9. Gerner T, Myren J, Larsen S. Premedication in upper gastrointestinal endoscopy. *Scand J Gastroenterol* 1983; 18: 925–928.
10. Taylor I, Duthie HL, Cumberland DC, Smallwood R. Glucagon and the colon. *Gut* 1975; 16: 973–978.
11. Chowdhury AR, Lorber SH. Effect of glucagon on cholecystokinin and Prostigmin-induced motor activity of the distal colon and rectum in humans. *Gastroenterology* 1975; 68: 875.
12. Chowdhury AR, Dinoso VP, Lorber SH. Characterization of a hyperactive segment at the rectosigmoid junction. *Gastroenterology* 1976; 71: 584–588.
13. Chowdhury AR, Lorber SH. Effects of glucagon and secretin on food- or morphine-induced motor activity of the distal colon, rectum, and anal sphincter. *Dig Dis* 1977; 22: 775–780.
14. Fujita K *et al.* Manometric study on colonic intraluminal pressure using the endoscopic method. *Gastroenterol Endosc* 1978; 21: 857.

DISCUSSION

Nikolov   Professor Takemoto, I believe you have mentioned that anticholinergic drugs are contraindicated in patients with prostatic hypertrophy. Have you used glucagon in these patients?

Takemoto   Yes I have. Actually, the administration of glucagon is not contraindicated in patients with glaucoma, prostatic hypertrophy or other conditions in which anticholinergic agents should not be given. Therefore, when we examine those patients we do use glucagon.

Carr-Locke   Professor Takemoto, tell me, was the first study you mentioned an open trial or was it a placebo-controlled trial?

Takemoto   It was an open trial.

Vilardell   We have used glucagon mostly in colonoscopy where we have observed that its administration occasionally produces side effects such as nausea or vomiting, and sometimes even a diarrhoeal flush in the bowel which disturbs the performance of colonoscopy. Would you comment on these problems or side effects please?

Takemoto   As far as nausea is concerned, it can be avoided to a great extent by decreasing the dose of glucagon or by giving it slowly. As a matter of fact, Abell and Malagelada (Abell TL, Malagelada JR. *Gastroenterology* 1985; 88: 1932–1940) have recently shown that there is a direct relationship between glucagon-induced gastric dysrhythmias and nausea and vomiting in healthy volunteers and, furthermore, they showed that the frequency of nausea episodes was higher in subjects receiving the larger doses of glucagon. On the other hand, diarrhoea, or rather the presence of liquid faeces in the colon lumen, is probably more the consequence of an insufficient cleansing of the colon than to an effect of glucagon.

Vilardell   It has been mentioned here that glucagon might decrease oesophageal motility and probably produce relaxation of the smooth muscle, and it has just occurred to me, even though it has nothing to do with endoscopy, that glucagon might be of help in patients with conditions which are related to oesophageal diffuse spasm. Do you agree with this?

Takemoto   Well yes, glucagon has been found to decrease the elevated resting pressure of the lower oesophageal sphincter of patients with achalasia, but its use as a therapeutic agent in this condition is rather limited. However, it has been suggested that glucagon can be used in practice when introducing catheters, specially in the pneumatic dilation of the cardia (Siewert R, Früh E, Waldeck F. *Dtsch Med Wschr* 1973; 98: 2045–2046) and it has also proved to relieve oesophageal spasm which can sometimes be seen as a complication or a consequence of β-adrenergic overdose and which may render impossible either the insertion or removal of an orogastric lavage tube. We all know that with the increasing range of therapeutic applicability and expanding availability of β-adrenergic antagonists, the risk of drug overdose has increased, and this potential complication should always be kept in mind.

Carr-Locke   Perhaps I could comment on that suggestion. I think that we are up against a problem of duration of action. During oesophageal manometry we can demonstrate that glucagon does have a relaxing effect, but in terms of therapy, we need agents that are much longer acting. That is why we tend to use long-acting nitrates which can be given orally, but I think that glucagon would work if we could give it for long enough.

Vilardell   In this respect I think that the situation has not changed in relation to the previous Workshop, since the oral route of administration for glucagon still remains to be clarified. Now changing to another point, I would like to raise a question: Might the differential diagnosis of chest pain in patients undergoing oesophageal studies be another field where glucagon could prove useful?

Skucas   I can give you some examples from personal observations. Occasionally, in radiology, in a patient with achalasia for instance, the question comes up of whether there is an underlying cancer which is producing the achalasia. In several of these patients we have used a dose of 0.5 mg of intravenous glucagon trying to get the lower oesophageal segment to distend in order to prove that there is no cancer, and invariably we have not been successful. So, essentially, we have abandoned this type of an approach.

Vilardell   Personally I cannot say that we have had that type of experience, but, to my knowledge, I think that your point is correct and, actually, we will be testing this for ourselves in the future.

6
Glucagon and the human biliary tree

D. L. CARR-LOCKE

INTRODUCTION

For many years following its discovery as a contaminant of insulin, glucagon was of little interest to gastroenterologists other than through its effects on glucose and glycogen metabolism. It is only relatively recently that the influences of glucagon on gastrointestinal motility, pancreatic and biliary secretion, and biliary motility have been realized, and it is these latter actions in man which are considered in this chapter. The relationship between glucagon and the human biliary tree will be discussed with respect to bile secretion, gallbladder motility, sphincter of Oddi motility and its clinical application in these areas insofar as this is not covered in other contributions to this workshop.

It is important to appreciate that when animal studies are quoted to support a particular effect of glucagon, these should be interpreted in the context of known or unknown species differences and the difficulties in extrapolating results to man. In addition, it is often the case that little regard is given to the precise dosage of glucagon administered by intravenous bolus or infusion with respect to its likely physiological or pharmacological effects. It seems that in man a physiological response in the biliary tract may be achieved by an infusion rate of up to $0.3\,\mu g\,kg^{-1}h^{-1}$ and that perhaps all bolus doses and infusions greater than $1.0\,\mu g\,kg^{-1}h^{-1}$ produce pharmacological effects and are not therefore necessarily relevant to normal human physiology.

BILE SECRETION

Mechanisms

Current views of bile secretion involve two mechanisms, one dependent on bile acid secretion and the other independent of bile acid secretion[1]. The basolateral membrane of the hepatocyte maintains a sodium-potassium ATPase system which has important implications for the transfer of bile acids and other organic anions from the hepatic sinusoids into the hepatocyte and thence across the canalicular membrane and into the bile canaliculus itself[2]. Independent of this is the secretion of water, bicarbonate, other anions and electrolytes into the bile canaliculus without the need for bile acid transfer and it is this aspect of bile secretion which may be under some control by peptide hormones[3]. It is also now clear that the tight junctions delimiting the bile canaliculus from the sinusoids are of paramount importance for the maintenance of electrolyte and voltage differences between canaliculus and cell[4].

Animal glucagon studies

Two animal models have been studied with respect to bile secretion and glucagon; there are considerable differences between them[5-11]. In the cat, Jansson et al.[5] have shown no effect of glucagon on hepatic bile flow at any dosage used. In contrast, several studies[4-10] have shown a significant effect in the dog model and three[6-8] have used physiological infusion rates from 0.03 to 0.18 $\mu g\,kg^{-1}h^{-1}$ when there was increased bile flow without change in either bile acid secretion or bicarbonate. This effect was not blocked by infusion of somatostatin nor cholinergic blockade. These studies also showed a reduced cholesterol and phospholipid output independent of these other phenomena. Unlike secretin[11,12], the choleretic action of glucagon seems to be independent of water and bicarbonate output and thus is probably a direct effect on the hepatocyte rather than through an intermediary peptide or other mechanism. Pharmacological doses of glucagon in the cholecystectomized dog[11] showed dramatic increases in bile flow of up to three times basal with increased electrolyte content and bile acid output but these effects are quite distinct from those seen at physiological levels.

Human glucagon studies

In man, accurate measurement of bile flow has only been possible in the cholecystectomized patient where a T-tube is present[13-17]. The study by Dyck and Janowitz[13] showed an effect of glucagon given in very small bolus doses and clearly showed a significant change in bile volume of 155% of control secretion without effect on electrolyte concentration after 0.5 $\mu g\,kg^{-1}$. This attained 169% after 1.0 μg kg^{-1} and was not further enhanced by 5.0 nor 10 μg kg^{-1} doses. In contrast, Jarrett and Bell[14] using 1 mg intravenous glucagon, given as a bolus, showed the choleretic effect in a patient being infused with the radiographic contrast medium iotroxamide (Figure 6.1). It is interesting to note that the increase in bile flow of less than 1 ml min^{-1} with this dose of glucagon is very similar to that achieved with much smaller doses and it is tempting to speculate that the stimulation of bile flow in response to glucagon in man has a maximum value achieved with very small doses which might conceivably be a physiological response. The effect of glucagon on bile composition in man is not as clear cut as in the dog model with reports of both unchanged hepatic bile constituents[13, 17] and increased electrolyte output[10, 11], although all probably represent pharmacological responses.

Thus, glucagon affects bile secretion in man by increasing the bile acid-independent fraction, but the mechanism is still not clear and whether or not this has physiological significance remains an open question.

GALLBLADDER MOTILITY

The assessment of gallbladder motility has been retarded by lack of an accurate means of measurement of gallbladder contraction and proportional emptying and filling. The traditional methods of oral cholecystography and ultrasound examinations have severe limitations and merely reflect overall changes in gallbladder volume. Perfusion studies using such non-absorbed molecules as polyethylene glycol and indocyanine green also tend to assess net changes by recovery of molecules from the duodenal lumen when used alone. Recent developments of isotope scanning techniques using such agents as ^{99m}Tc-HIDA and ^{75}SeHCAT have provided much more information about gallbladder filling and emptying and using both isotopes simultaneously or ^{99m}Tc-HIDA with indocyanine green has allowed a much more detailed analysis of these events[18, 19]. One of the current concepts is of the gallbladder behaving like a bellows with a series of filling and emptying movements taking place (perhaps simultaneous with phases of sphincter of Oddi activity), superimposed on the more traditional concept of a slow net filling phase and storage of bile followed by a more rapid net emptying phase at the time of food stimulation[20]. The effect of glucagon on gallbladder motility seems to vary widely amongst animal models with no effect being shown in the cat[5] and guinea-pig[21] but a fall in intraluminal gallbladder pressure and relaxation of the gallbladder wall in the dog[9, 22].

There are very few studies in man but that by Chernish et al.[23] using a large 2 mg intravenous bolus dose of glucagon showed relaxation of the gallbladder shadow on oral cholecystography while no effect was seen by Cameron et al.[24] with strips of human gallbladder muscle studied in vitro. There are no

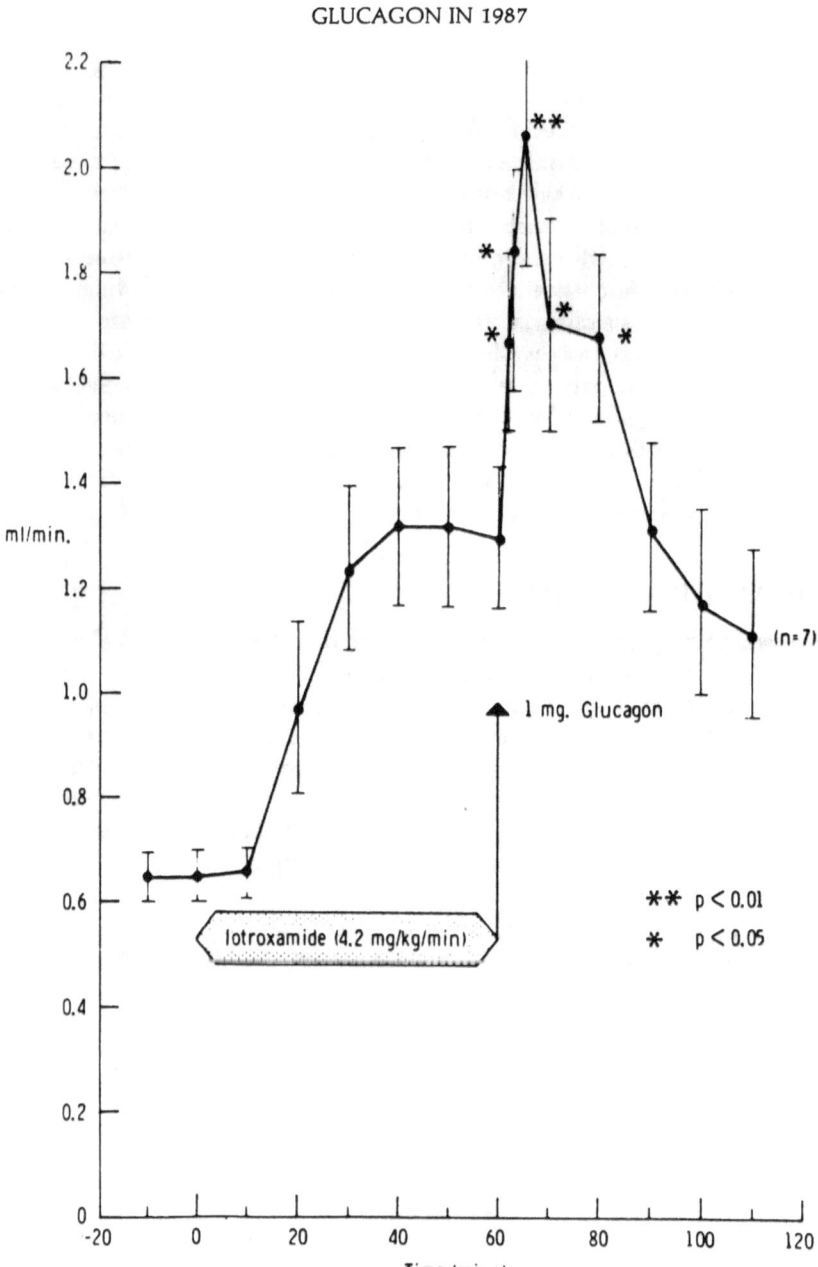

Figure 6.1 Graph showing effect of 1 mg intravenous glucagon on mean bile flow in seven postoperative T-tube patients given a 1h intravenous infusion of iotroxamide ($4.2 \, mg \, kg^{-1} \, min^{-1}$) (Reproduced from ref. 14 by kind permission of *Clinical Radiology* and the author)

studies using physiological doses of glucagon available and this question remains unanswered.

SPHINCTER OF ODDI MOTILITY

This year, 1987, is the centenary of Oddi's classical description of the sphincter which now bears his name[25]. Anatomical details of this sphincteric zone show a complex structure of interdigitating muscle fibres[26] which although important for understanding does not allow a clear picture of physiology and pathophysiology when considering its function. Radiographically it is possible to see the function of the sphincteric zone (Figure 6.2) as an opening and closing channel in the terminal portions of both common bile duct and pancreatic duct. In addition, it is possible to visualize a sphincteric zone confined to the pancreatic duct alone (Figure 6.3) suggesting that in functional terms there are two areas of sphincteric activity, one surrounding the terminal common bile duct and the other the terminal pancreatic duct close to the duodenal papilla with some sharing of fibres at their confluence[26].

Endoscopic manometry

Study of this small area in man has been extremely difficult until the advent, very recently, of direct methods of access. Previous techniques depended on indirect access intra-operatively or through T-tubes in post-operative patients and were of questionable relevance to normal human physiology.

The ability to cannulate the duodenal papilla endoscopically has not only allowed the development of diagnostic and therapeutic procedures but has also allowed the investigator to pass manometry devices across the papilla and into the two ductal systems[27]. Details of the technique of endoscopic manometry have been well described[27, 28] by several centres and all involved in this work are now able to demonstrate basal and phasic pressure profiles from the sphincteric zone. Although our group initially used a moderately compliant syringe pump perfusion system[26], we, like others, changed to the low compliance pneumohydraulic capillary infusion system introduced some eight years ago[27]. Our current practice is to use a triple lumen catheter perfused with sterile water at $0.3\ ml\ min^{-1}$ which provides a pressure rise rate of $200\ mmHg\ s^{-1}$ and fidelity far in excess of that required for following phasic recordings from the sphincter of Oddi. The procedure is carried out in a lightly sedated subject, lying prone, with a standard duodenoscope placed opposite to the duodenal papilla through which the manometry catheter may be passed and then connected to the perfusing and recording systems. The use of a triple lumen catheter with 10 mm spacing of the distal side-openings facilitates measurement of ductal, sphincteric and duodenal pressures concurrently (Figure

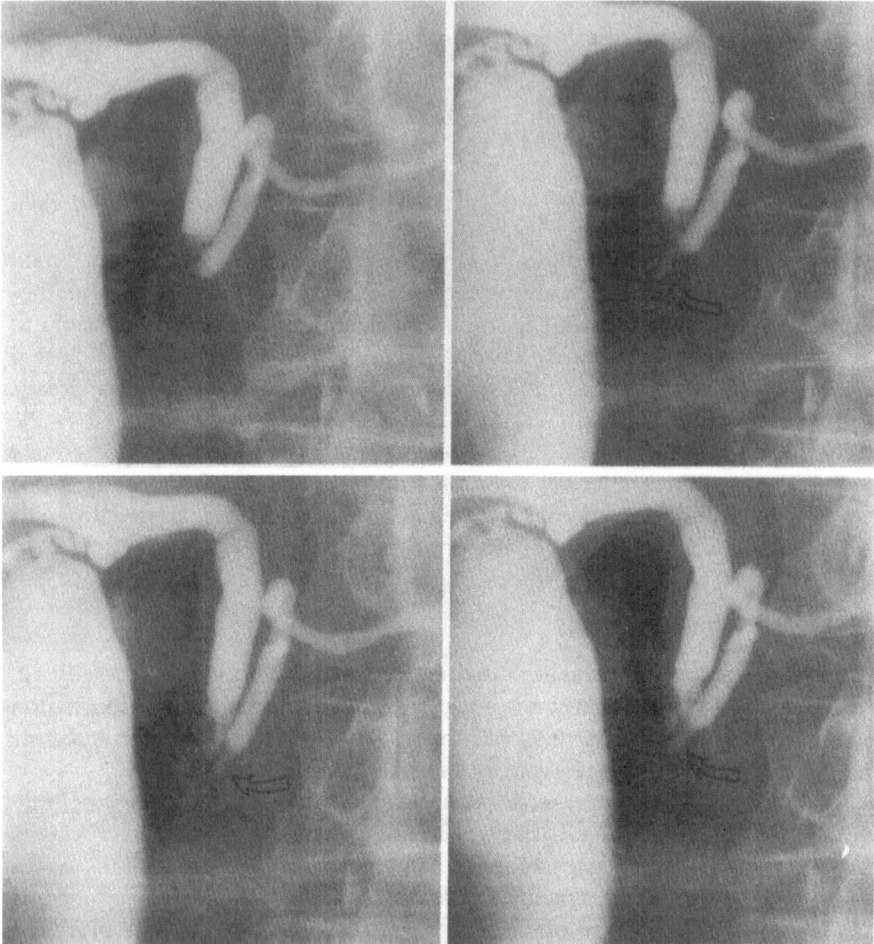

Figure 6.2 Radiograph series following ERCP showing closed and open phases of pancreatic sphincter (open arrow) and biliary sphincter (closed arrow) components of sphincter of Oddi

6.4). The extraction of mean ductal pressure, phasic basal, peak and amplitude pressures and wave frequency and duration have been internationally agreed[29]. There is still some controversy, however, about whether or not it is valid to express manometric results as different when station pull-through recordings are taken from either the pancreatic or bile duct, although our group has always reported these values separately[27, 30].

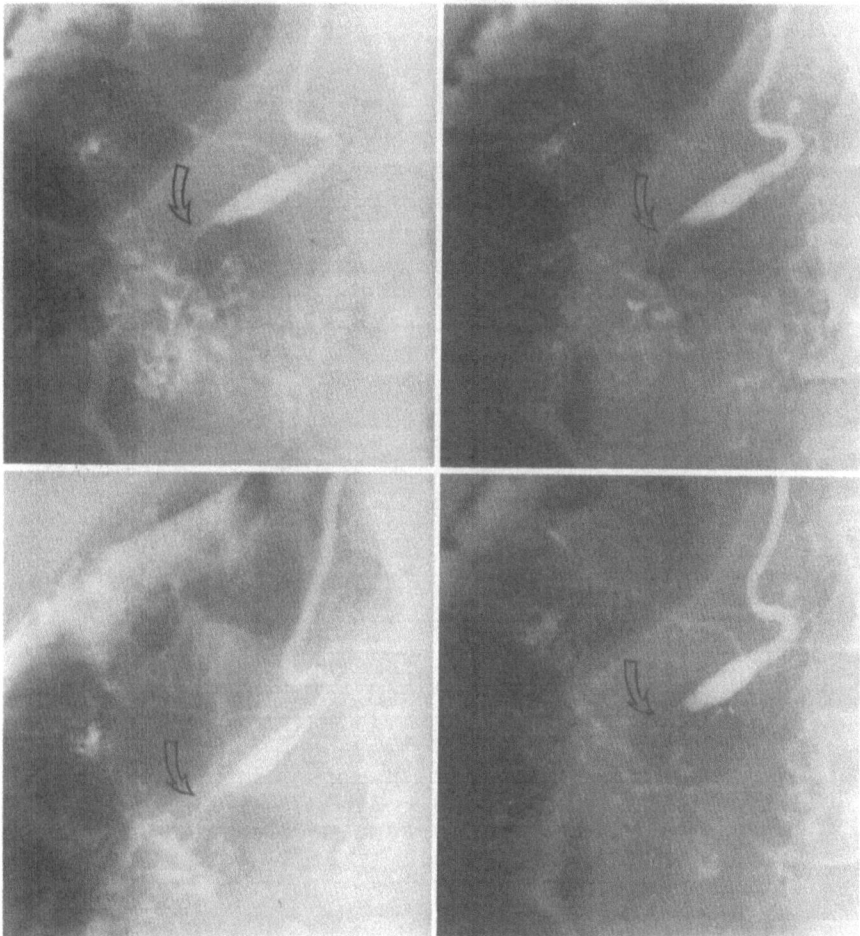

Figure 6.3. Radiograph series following ERCP showing pancreatic sphincter (open arrow)

Physiology of glucagon

The published literature on the effects of glucagon on the sphincter of Oddi principally concerns itself with large doses (0.4–1.0 mg) producing pharmacological actions either when given intravenously, in man[31–33] or animals[9, 22, 34, 35], or topically in man by direct application onto the papilla[36] (as has also been found with glucagon 1–21-peptide[37–40]). The aim of one study, however[31], was to assess the sphincter of Oddi in relation to very small doses of glucagon which might simulate the physiological state. Studying eleven male (including the author) and nine female normal volunteers, endoscopic

73

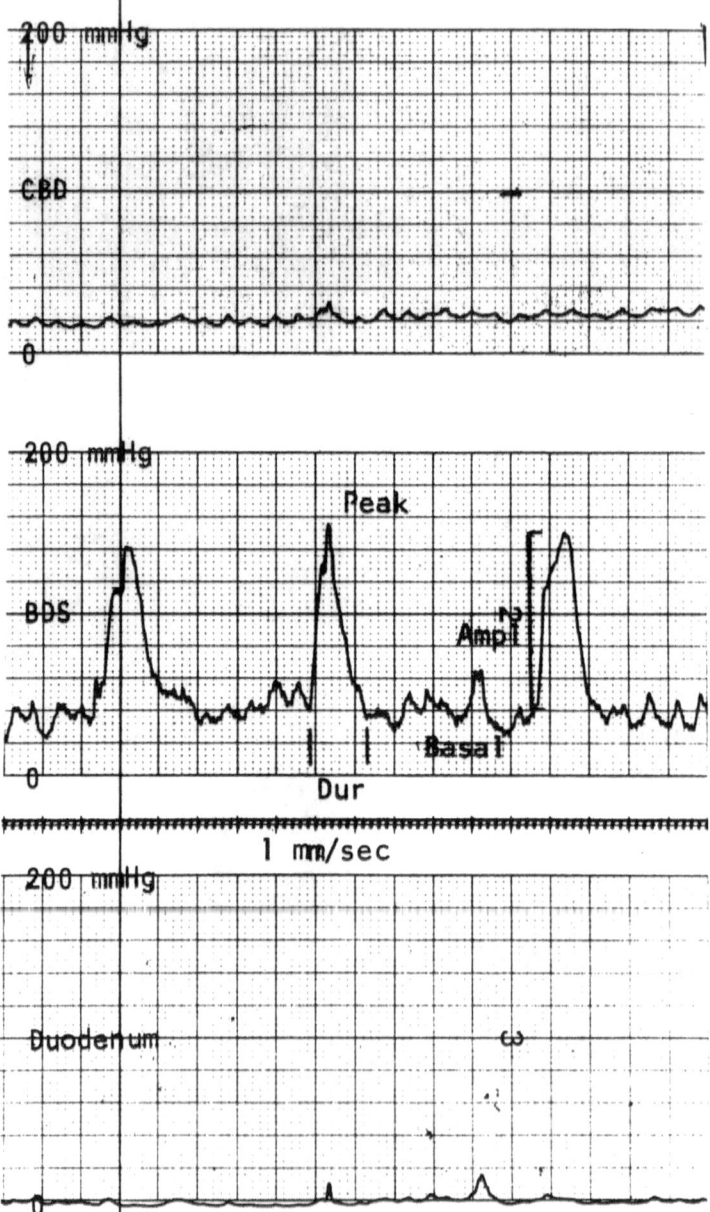

Figure 6.4 Tracing from triple lumen endoscopic manometry catheter showing pressures in common bile duct (CBD, upper trace), duodenum (lower trace) and bile duct sphincter (BDS) zone (middle trace) with peak, basal and amplitude values marked

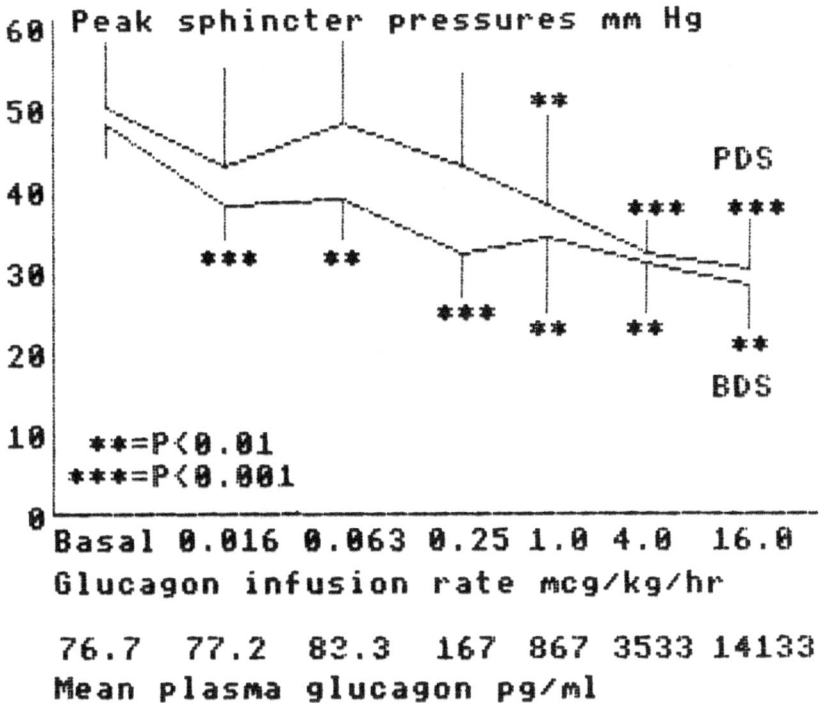

Figure 6.5 Graph showing effects of increasing glucagon infusion dosage on peak pancreatic duct sphincter (PDS) and bile duct sphincter (BDS) pressures (redrawn from ref. 31)

manometry was accomplished during saline infusion and then repeated during a stepwise increasing dose of glucagon from 0.016 to 16.0 μg hg^{-1}h^{-1} with monitoring of plasma glucagon concentrations. The three lowest infusion rates from 0.016 to 0.25 μg hg^{-1}h^{-1} were found to produce plasma levels within the physiological range contemporaneous with which bile duct sphincter pressures were significantly lowered without effect on the pancreatic sphincter (Figure 6.5). Only at supraphysiological doses were pancreatic pressures and both ductal and duodenal pressures lowered and phasic wave frequency and duration reduced. These findings were subsequently confirmed in a separate study when glucagon was infused at 0.016 μg hg^{-1}h^{-1} for 10 min and then stopped, during which endoscopic manometry continued and showed falls in bile duct sphincter pressure followed by a return to basal values[31].

Pharmacology of glucagon

The effect of glucagon given as a bolus dose of 1 mg was also assessed[31] as this was of interest in relation to its use in radiological procedures and therapeutics. This produces a dramatic change in plasma glucagon concentration with a peak in excess of 200 000 pg ml^{-1} and a half-life of 8.5 min. The effects on both pancreatic and bile duct sphincters were equal, with relaxation manifesting as a reduction in wave frequency and duration to less than half the initial rates and falls in amplitude and, to a lesser extent, basal pressure, with reduction in ductal pressures and relaxation of the duodenum. These phenomena have been disputed by other workers and a further study was therefore undertaken more recently (Carr-Locke, D.L. and Bentley, S., 1986, unpublished data) to clarify whether or not these observations were genuine or artefactual. Following an initial manometric recording from the bile duct sphincter either 1 mg of glucagon or an equivalent volume of saline was given intravenously in a double-blind manner and after 3–5 min manometric recordings from the bile duct sphincter were repeated. The investigator was then asked to classify all those traces thought to have been associated with glucagon and all those with placebo and, as shown in Figure 6.6, all were correctly identified. There were no changes in any parameter measured in the saline group but dramatic falls in phasic pressures and loss of phasic activity occurred in all receiving glucagon.

The precise cellular mechanism linking glucagon with its 'spasmolytic' effects on gastrointestinal smooth muscle remains to be elucidated but animal studies[22] have failed to show any interference with the actions of glucagon on the sphincter of Oddi by the concurrent administration of an adrenergic β-antagonist such as propranolol, an a-adrenergic antagonist such as phenoxybenzamine, a muscarinic blocker such as atropine or a ganglion-blocking agent such as pentolinium.

One further action of glucagon is worthy of mention. As an inhibitor of gastrointestinal motility glucagon would seem to have opposing effects to opiates[41, 42], characterized by the actions of morphine. We therefore studied the influence of glucagon on the sphincter of Oddi already stimulated by a single intravenous injection of 5 mg morphine (Carr-Locke, D.L. and Gregg, J.A. 1979, unpublished data). Figure 6.7 shows the characteristic 12 cycles per min phasic activity induced by morphine which after 2 min following injection of 1 mg glucagon slows to near normal activity. This suggests that morphine and glucagon either share a common receptor site or some common pathway of smooth muscle cell control perhaps through their known effects on intracellular cyclic nucleotides.

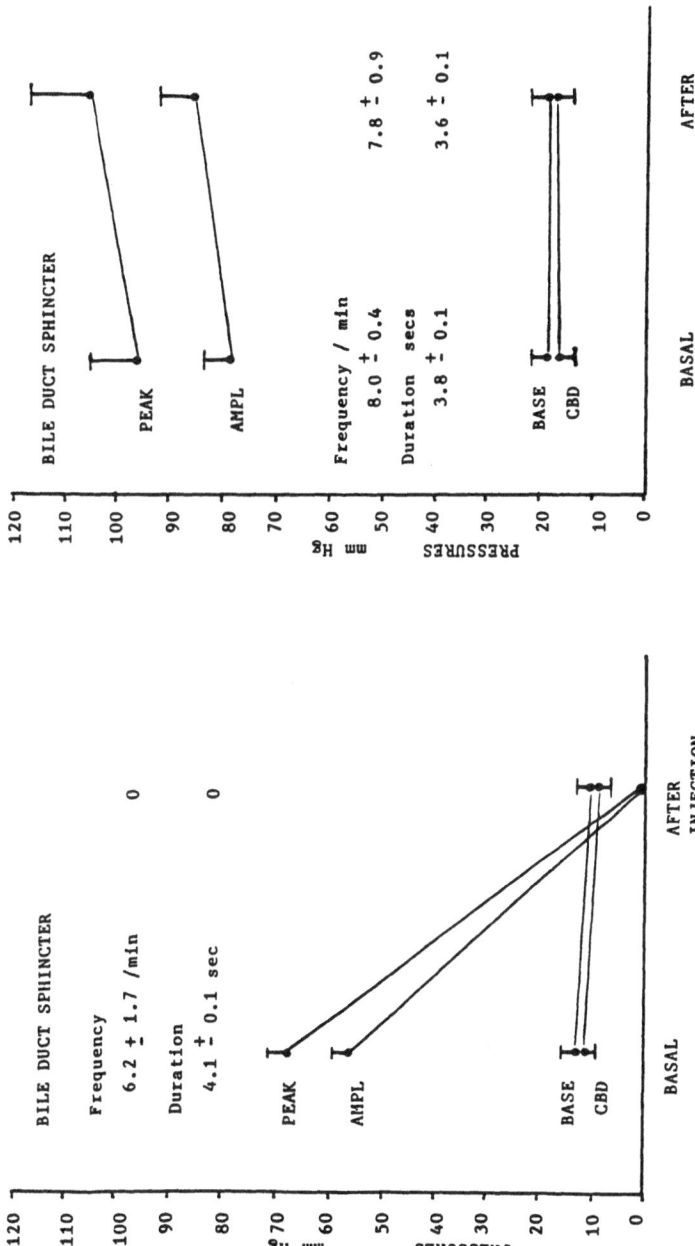

Figure 6.6 Graphs showing results of double-blind assessment of 1 mg glucagon given as an intravenous bolus in 20 subjects undergoing endoscopic manometry of the bile duct sphincter with all test injections correctly classified as glucagon (left) or placebo (right)

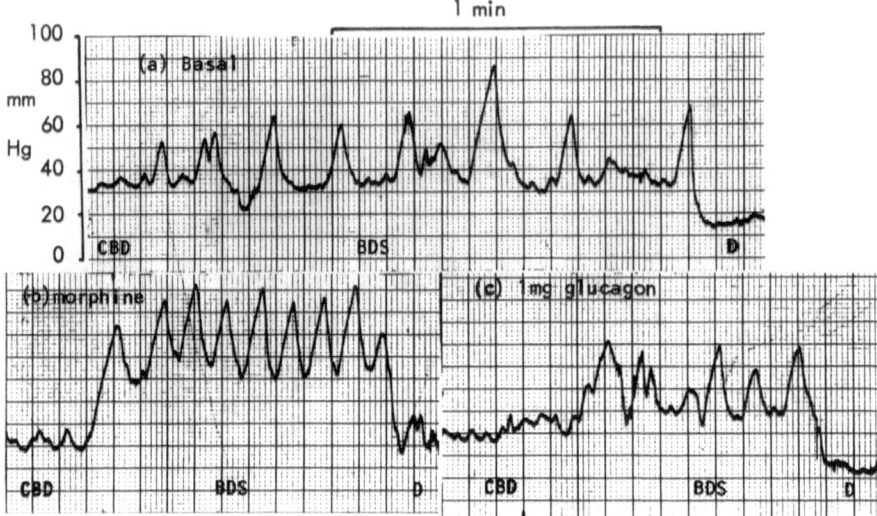

Figure 6.7 Three endoscopic manometry traces from the same subject in sequence showing common bile duct (CBD), duodenal (D) and bile duct sphincter (BDS) pressures under (a) basal conditions, (b) after 5 mg intravenous morphine and (c) 2 min after 1 mg intravenous glucagon given at (b)

CLINICAL APPLICATIONS

Clinical application of glucagon with respect to its biliary actions falls into diagnostic and therapeutic categories employing both its effects on bile secretion and motility.

Diagnostic applications

Ultrasound

With increasing sophistication of real-time ultrasound in the investigation of suspected biliary disorders, the role of glucagon is likely to become more limited. There is occasionally, however, a need to produce temporary cessation of all local gastrointestinal movement in order to enhance ultrasonic views of the bile duct and gallbladder and an intravenous or intramuscular injection of 1 mg glucagon will achieve this[43, 44].

Cholecystography

Despite the observed relaxation effect of glucagon on the human gallbladder[23] during oral cholecystography, this has not become a standard technique and finds little application in the routine investigation of gallbladder symptoms.

When used during intravenous cholangiography (*vide infra*) the combined effects of choleresis and gallbladder atony may fortuitously further enhance opacification[14].

Intravenous infusion cholangiography

Optimal success of intravenous cholangiography depends on the excretion of an iodine-containing contrast medium in adequate concentrations within bile to provide a radiographic image[45]. The known choleretic action of glucagon, affecting the bile acid-independent fraction of bile secretion, might tend to dilute any radiographic contrast already present in the bile duct or being excreted simultaneously, unless this agent were in some way also involved in the choleretic stimulation process when opacification might actually be increased. These opposing possibilities, which are presumed to be due to differences in behaviour between different contrast media, may provide the explanations for the conflicting findings of enhanced[14, 46, 47] and impaired[48] visualization of the bile duct during infusion cholangiography.

Percutaneous transhepatic cholangiography

Glucagon has been reported as being of some benefit during percutaneous cholangiography[46, 49] but the advantages are not clear cut and there has been no move to incorporate glucagon as standard practice for this procedure in radiology departments.

Operative cholangiography and radiomanometry

Glucagon has been recommended for relaxing the terminal segment of the common bile duct and for the relief of sphincter of Oddi 'spasm' which may be present during operative cholangiography as a result of instrumentation and the side-effects of narcotics[41, 42, 50]. A controlled study[51], with 1 mg glucagon against saline, assessed cholangiographic image quality and concluded that glucagon was superior in allowing adequate filling of all bile duct structures more often and more successfully than saline. The technique of operative radiomanometry has been of varied popularity in Europe and the USA but continues to be used in some interested centres for the detection of abnormal biliary dynamics due to residual calculi or pathology at the level of the papilla. Several enthusiasts have suggested that glucagon is of considerable benefit[52, 53] for facilitating the examination by reducing filling, resting and perfusion pressures and increasing flow which especially enables the operator to distinguish a temporary motility abnormality from a pathological obstruction.

Endoscopic retrograde cholangiography

It is standard practice during endoscopic retrograde cholangiography (ERCP) to induce temporary paralysis of the duodenum in order to allow adequate visualization of the papilla and facilitate cannulation prior to the injection of radiographic contrast or a subsequent therapeutic procedure. Although an anticholinergic drug such as hyoscine-N-butylbromide is commonly employed for this purpose, there are disadvantages to its use and an alternative without side-effects would be preferable. Glucagon given intravenously in doses from 0.5 to 2.0 mg has been assessed in this context in three studies[54-56] and was found equally effective compared to butropium[54] and hyoscine[55] and superior to saline[56] in success of performing ERCP but was accompanied by fewer adverse effects. In order to avoid the metabolic consequences and induction of nausea associated with pharmacological doses of glucagon the author has recently completed a double-blind study (Carr-Locke, D.L., 1986, unpublished data) in forty patients undergoing ERCP with glucagon 1–21-peptide which is known to retain the spasmolytic properties of the parent hormone[39, 40] and also have the desired effects on duodenum and sphincter of Oddi[37, 38]. Despite these demonstrable actions, in practice glucagon 1–21-peptide at a dose of 4 mg given as an intravenous bolus did not improve visualization of the papilla nor the ease of cannulation during ERCP and endoscopic sphincterotomy compared with placebo and cannot therefore be recommended at the dosage studied as an alternative to current procedures.

Therapeutic applications

Biliary pain

Several open[57, 58] and controlled[59-61] clinical studies have now shown that glucagon or its 1–21-peptide[62] given as an initial intravenous bolus and, if necessary, followed by a continuous infusion of up to 1 mg per 4 h, will alleviate the pain of biliary disease due to cholelithiasis and/or choledocholithiasis without significant side-effects other than the expected degree of hyperglycaemia.

Choledocholithiasis

There are no controlled trials of glucagon for the relief of calculous obstruction of the bile duct but it has been used to expedite passage of stones retained after biliary surgery when a T-tube is present with some success[57, 59, 63, 64] and is perhaps always worth attempting before proceeding to more invasive techniques of stone extraction.

Choleretic therapy

The choleretic effect of glucagon given in supraphysiological doses has been put to clinical advantage in three recent studies[65-67]. Kobayashi *et al.*[65] looked at the accelerated reduction of hyperbilirubinaemia induced by glucagon following percutaneous transhepatic drainage of the biliary system, Constantopoulos *et al.*[66] also detected a significant fall in hyperbilirubinaemia in neonates so affected, and so avoided phototherapy in many, and Watanabe *et al.*[67], in a preliminary report, suggested that glucagon might prevent the cholangitis complicating Kasai's operation performed for biliary atresia.

CONCLUSIONS

Glucagon now has a well-established profile of effects on bile secretion and biliary motility in man although detailed mechanisms have still to be elucidated. Clinical application of these actions has become commonplace during radiological and endoscopic procedures and its use as a therapeutic agent for biliary pain and as a choleretic is increasing. Further research into shorter peptides derived from the parent hormone is required in order to separate the metabolic from its other effects in the hope that a clinically useful agent will become available for diagnostic and therapeutic procedures devoid of significant adverse properties.

References

1. Erlinger S. Physiology of bile secretion. In: Bouchier IAD, Allan RN, Hodgson HJF, Keighley MRB, eds. *Textbook of Gastroenterology*. London: Baillière Tindall 1984: 1380–1389.
2. Boyer JL. New concepts of mechanisms of hepatocyte bile formation. *Physiol Rev* 1980; 60: 303–326.
3. Moseley RH, Boyer JL. Mechanisms of electrolyte transport in the liver and their functional significance. *Semin Liver Dis* 1985; 5: 122–135.
4. Boyer JL. Tight junctions in normal and cholestatic liver: does the paracellular pathway have functional significance? *Hepatology* 1983; 3: 614–617.
5. Jansson R, Steen G, Svanik J. A comparison of glucagon, gastric inhibitory peptide, and secretin on gallbladder function, formation of bile and pancreatic secretion in the cat. *Scand J Gastroenterol* 1978; 13: 919–925.
6. Garberoglio CA, Bickerstaff KI, Baker AL, Moossa AR. Is glucagon a choleretic hormone at physiological blood levels? *Am J Surg* 1982; 143: 61–66.
7. Schirmer BD, Kortz WJ, Miller RM, Jones RS. Glucagon lowers biliary cholesterol output at physiological doses. *Gastroenterology* 1982; 82: 1171.
8. Bickerstaff KI, Garberoglio CA, Baker AL, Moossa AR. Hormonal control of biliary lipid secretion in dogs. *Ann Surg* 1983; 198: 168–171.
9. Lin TM, Spray GF. Effect of pentagastrin, cholecystokinin, caerulein, and glucagon on the choledochal resistance and bile flow in conscious dog. *Gastroenterology* 1969; 56: 1178.
10. Kaminsky DL, Ruwart MJ, Jellinek M. Effect of glucagon on secretin-stimulated bile flow. *Am J Physiol* 1975; 229: 1480–1485.
11. Morris TQ, Sardi GF, Bradley SE. Character of glucagon induced choleresis. *Fed Proc* 1967; 26: 774.
12. Khedis A, Dumont M, Duval M, Erlinger S. Influence of glucagon on canalicular bile production in the dog. *Biomedicine* 1974; 21: 176–181.

13. Dyck K, Janowitz HD. Effect of glucagon on hepatic bile secretion in man. *Gastroenterology* 1971; 60: 400–404.
14. Jarrett LN, Bell GD. Effect of intravenous glucagon on the biliary secretion of a cholangiographic agent in man. *Clin Radiol* 1980; 31: 657–661.
15. Dura K, Wedrichowicz A, Rucinski M. Effect of glucagon on bile lipids. *Polski Tygod Lekar* 1976; 31: 433–435.
16. Levine RA, Hall RC. Cyclic AMP in secretin choleresis. Evidence for a regulatory role in man and baboons but not in dogs. *Gastroenterology* 1976; 70: 537–544.
17. Poulantzas J, Polymeropoulos T, Papastamatiou L, Vachiotis P, Liassidis E. Biliary secretion after intravenous administration of glucagon. Presented at the 20th Biennial World Congress of the Internat Coll Surg, Athens 1976. Oxford: Excerpta Medica, 1976: 625.
18. Sarva RP, Schreiner DP, Van Thiel D, Yingvorapant N. Gallbladder function, methods for measuring filling and emptying. *J. Nucl Med* 1985; 26: 140–144.
19. Jazrawi RP, Lanzini A, Britten A, Meller ST, Northfield TC. Dynamics of gallbladder function and of the enterohepatic circulation studies by a γ-labelled bile acid. *Clin Sci* 1984; 66: 10P.
20. Lanzini A, Jazrawi RJ, Northfield TC. Does the gallbladder function as a pump or as a bellows? *Gut* 1983; 24: A475.
21. Vagne M, Troitskaja V. Effect of secretin, glucagon and VIP on gallbladder contraction. *Digestion* 1976; 14: 62–67.
22. Lin TM. Actions of gastrointestinal hormones and related peptides on the motor function of the biliary tract. *Gastroenterology* 1975; 69: 1006–1022.
23. Chernish SM, Miller RE, Rosenak BD, Scholz NE. Effect of glucagon on size of visualised human gallbladder before and after a fat meal. *Gastroenterology* 1982; 62: 1218–1226.
24. Cameron AJ, Phillips SF, Summerskill WHJ. Effect of cholecystokinin, gastrin, secretin and glucagon on human gallbladder muscle *in vitro. Proc Soc Exp Biol Med* 1969; 131: 149–154.
25. Oddi R. D'une exposition a sphincter speciale de l'ouverture du canal choledoque. *Arch Ital Biol* 1887; 8: 317–322.
26. Boyden EA. The sphincter of Oddi in man and certain representative mammals. *Surgery* 1937; 1: 25–37.
27. Carr-Locke DL, Gregg JA. Endoscopic manometry of pancreatic and biliary sphincter zones in man. Basal results in healthy volunteers. *Dig Dis Sci* 1981; 26: 7–15.
28. Geenen JE, Hogan WJ, Dodds WJ, Stewart ET, Arndorfer RC. Intraluminal pressure recording from the human sphincter of Oddi. *Gastroenterology* 1980; 78: 317–324.
29. International Workshop on Sphincter of Oddi Manometry, Rome, 1985. *Ital J Gastroenterol* 1986; 18: 31–45.
30. Carr-Locke DL, Gregg JA, Chey WY. Effects of exogenous secretin on pancreatic and biliary ductal and sphincteric pressures in man demonstrated by endoscopic manometry and correlation with plasma secretin levels. *Dig Dis Sci* 1985; 30: 909–917.
31. Carr-Locke DL, Gregg, JA, Aoki TT. Effects of exogenous glucagon on pancreatic and biliary ductal and sphincteric pressures in man demonstrated by endoscopic manometry and correlation with plasma glucagon. *Dig Dis Sci* 1983; 62: 312–320.
32. Carr-Locke DL. Effects of gut peptides on human sphincter of Oddi function. *Ital J Gastroenterol* 1986; 18: 43–45.
33. Rey JF, Corallo J, Lombart J, Pangtay-Tea J. The use of endoscopic manometry to demonstrate the effect of glucagon on the sphincter of Oddi. In, Picazo J, Ed. *Glucagon in Gastroenterology and Hepatology.* Lancaster: MTP Press, 1982: 99–114.
34. Sarles JC, Delecourt P, Castello H, Gaeta L, Nacchiero M, Amoros JP, Devaux MA, Awad R. Action of gastrointestinal hormones on the myoelectrical activity of the sphincter of Oddi in the living rabbit. *Regul Peptides* 1981; 2: 113–124.
35. Behar J. Comparative pharmacological characteristics of the lower esophageal sphincter (LES) and the sphincter of Oddi (SO) in the cat *in vivo. Dig Dis Sci* 1980; 25: 720.
36. Ponce J, Sala T, Pertejo V, Pina R, Berenguer J. Effect of glucagon applied topically in the duodenum on the motor activity of the sphincter of Oddi. *Acta Endosc* 1983; 13: 131–138.
37. Rey JF, Greff M, Picazo J. Relaxation of the sphincter of Oddi by glucagon-(1–21)-peptide applied locally to the periampullary mucosa. *Gut* 1985; 26: 78.

38. Rey JF, Greff M, Picazo J. Glucagon-(1–21)-peptide. Study of its action on sphincter of Oddi function by endoscopic manometry. *Dig Dis Sci* 1986; 31: 355–360.
39. Diamant B, Jorgensen KD, Weis JU. Structure–activity relationship for the spasmolytic action of glucagon. In: Picazo J, Ed. *Glucagon in Gastroenterology and Hepatology.* Lancaster: MTP Press, 1982: 25–36.
40. Jorgensen KD, Weis JU, Diamant B. Dissociation of the spasmolytic and metabolic effects of glucagon. *Eur J Pharmacol* 1983; 90: 315–323.
41. Jones RM, Fiddian-Green R, Knight PR. Narcotic-induced choledochoduodenal sphincter spasm reversed by glucagon. *Anesth Analg* 1980; 59: 946–947.
42. McCammon RL, Stoelting R, Madura JA. Reversal of fentanyl-induced spasm of the sphincter of Oddi. *Surg Gynecol Obstet* 1983; 156: 329–334.
43. Pon MS, Cooperberg PL. Oral water and intravenous glucagon – to aid ultrasonic visualization of the common bile duct. *J Can Assoc Radiol* 1979; 30: 173–174.
44. Weighall SL, Wolfman NT, Watson N. The fluid-filled stomach: a new sonic window. *J Clin Ultrasound* 1979; 7: 353–356.
45. Carr-Locke DL. Diagnosis. In: Bateson MC, ed. *Gallstone Disease and its Management.* Lancaster: MTP Press, 1986: 71–113.
46. Canon P, Legge D. Glucagon as the hypotonic agent in cholangiography. *Clin Radiol* 1979; 30: 49–52.
47. Evans AF, Whitehouse GW. The effect of glucagon on infusion cholangiography. *Clin Radiol* 1979; 30: 499–506.
48. Jarrett LN, Doran J, Clifford K, Keane D, Knapp DR, Bell GD. Glucagon and infusion cholangiography. *Br J Radiol* 1982; 55: 269–271.
49. Mueller PR, Harbin WP, Ferrucci JT, Wittenberg J, van Sonnenberg E. Fine-needle transhepatic cholangiography: reflections after 450 cases. *Am J Roentgenol* 1981; 136: 85–90.
50. Bordley J, Olson JE. The use of glucagon in operative cholangiography. *Surg Gynecol Obstet* 1979; 149: 583–584.
51. Tabak CA, Tuxen PL, Bruce DL, Juler GL. Glucagon enhancement of cholangiography. A preliminary report. *Arch Surg* 1983; 118: 84–85.
52. Treffot MJ, Quilichini F, Vinson MF. Biliary surgery, radiomanometry and glucagon. In: Picazo J, ed. *Glucagon in Gastroenterology,* Lancaster: MTP Press, 1979: 87–94.
53. McCarthy JD. Biliary radiomanometry as an investigative tool in biliary tract disease. In: Picazo J, ed. *Glucagon in Gastroenterology,* Lancaster: MTP Press, 1979: 95–102.
54. Ueda N, Kohriyama E, Suzuki Y, Takai Y, Okamura K, Ishibashi M, Mizushima K, Namiki M. Usefulness of glucagon as premedication for endoscopic retrograde cholangiopancreatography. (Jap). *Gastroenterol Endosc* 1983; 25: 1500–1505.
55. Hannigan BF, Axon ATR, Avery S, Thompson RPH. Buscopan or glucagon for endoscopic cannulation of ampulla of Vater? *J Roy Soc Med* 1982; 75: 21–22.
56. Silvis SE, Vennes JA. The role of glucagon in endoscopic cholangiopancreatography. *Gastrointest Endosc* 1975; 21: 162–163.
57. Paul F. The role of glucagon in the treatment of biliary tract pathology. In: Picazo J, ed. *Glucagon in Gastroenterology.* Lancaster: MTP Press, 1979: 107–117.
58. Brandstatter G, Kratochvil P. Glucagon bei Gallenkoliken. *Therapiewoche* 1979; 29: 3362–3365.
59. Stower MJ, Foster GE, Hardcastle JD. A trial of glucagon in the treatment of painful biliary tract disease. *Br J Surg* 1982; 69: 591–592.
60. Hardcastle JD, Stower MJ, Foster GE. The use of glucagon in spastic disorders of the gastrointestinal tract. In: Picazo J, Ed. *Glucagon in Gastroenterology.* Lancaster: MTP Press, 1982: 115–127.
61. Grossi E, Broggini M, Quaranta M, Balestrino E. Different pharmacological approaches to the treatment of acute biliary colic. *Curr Ther Res* 1986; 40: 876–882.
62. Jacobson G, Nilsonn B, Nordgren CE, Selking O. Glucagon-(1–21)-peptide to prevent biliary colic pain. *Lancet* 1984; 2: 1149.
63. Doman DB, Ginsberg AL. Glucagon infusion therapy for biliary tree stones. *Gastroenterology* 1981; 80: 1137.
64. Latshaw RF, Kadir S, Witt WS, Kaufman SL, White RI. Glucagon-induced choledochal

sphincter relaxation: aid for expulsion of impacted calculi into the duodenum. *Am J Roentgenol* 1981; 137: 614–616.

65. Kobayashi M, Muto M, Shimada H, Kito F, Shinmyo K, Abe T, Kure H, Tsuchiya S. Effect of glucagon on hepatic bile in obstructive jaundice. (Jap). *Nippon Shokakibyo Gakki Zassui* 1982; 79: 952–955.
66. Constantopoulos A, Davakis M, Malamitsi-Pouchner A, Matsaniotis N. The effect of glucagon on serum bilirubin levels. *Cytobios* 1982; 35: 103–111.
67. Watanabe Y, Todani T, Kobayashi T, Fujii T, Arata A. Glucagon administration for the treatment of postoperative cholangitis after Kasai's operation – a preliminary report. *Z Kinderchir* 1983; 38: 83–87.

DISCUSSION

Nikolov   Dr Carr-Locke, are there any significant differences between the effect of glucagon on bile and bile components depending on whether the dose is a physiologic or a pharmacological one?

Carr-Locke   As I mentioned in my lecture, if one uses small doses of glucagon, the change in bile volume is independent of other changes. In other words, bile acid concentration does not change, sodium, potassium, calcium and magnesium do not change, phospholipid does not change, but cholesterol, for some strange reason, may actually fall. If one uses a very big dose of glucagon, then bile secretion, bile acid output, and sodium and potassium output may actually rise. So, indeed, these two effects may be different.

Nikolov   And, what about bilirubin?

Carr-Locke   That we do not know. The problem is that most of these studies have been done in non-jaundiced patients postoperatively; so, in other words, their plasma bilirubin levels are normal, and their hepatic bile bilirubin levels are likely to be normal, which makes it very difficult to detect any change. What would be much more interesting would be to do a study in jaundiced patients where perhaps we would be able to assess the clearance of bilirubin, which is what we are interested in. So, I really cannot answer your question.

Lefèbvre   Dr Carr-Locke, the species differences that you have shown are extremely important. In one of the books that I published, Diamant and Picazo reported studies done with different fragments of glucagon (Diamant B, Picazo J. In: Lefèbvre PJ, ed. *Handbook of Experimental Pharmacology. 66 II*. Berlin, Heidelberg, New York, Tokyo: Springer, 1983: 611–643). All these fragments were tested by some *in vitro* system using smooth muscle, and there were very promising compounds in these *in vitro* systems, but none of them prevailed, because those that were effective *in vitro* in the smooth muscle tissue of a particular animal, later proved not to be very active in man, and as you have seen, the reverse can also be true; you have shown a good example of glucagon acting in one system *in vivo* and not *in vitro*. So, I think that this question of species differences for the screening of the effects of glucagon and glucagon fragments is extremely important. Do you agree with this?

Carr-Locke   Absolutely, yes. Our experience with the 1–21 glucagon fragment is a good example of a situation where species differences have led us to use a substance in man which, unfortunately, does not seem to produce the effects that we expected, and that was because we were misled by the animal data.

Lefèbvre   I think this is a point which is completely ignored by many people. Now, to deal with the interesting finding by which glucagon reversed the effects of morphine and opiates (Jones RM, Fiddian-Green R, Knight PR. *Anaesth Analg* 1980; 59: 946–947), I find that this is an interesting theoretical aspect which may shed some light on the mechanism of action of glucagon, but in the case of an intense spasm of the Oddi sphincter, would you advise giving glucagon, or rather the antagonist naloxone for instance?

Carr-Locke   That is a very interesting question. It really depends on the clinical situation. If, for instance, one is considering the preoperative situation where something like fentanyl has been given during surgery one does not want to reverse the analgesic properties of it, but one does want to reverse the motility effects. So, it is therefore illogical to give naloxone, which would reverse both. One gives glucagon, which does not seem to reverse the analgesic effects. If, however, we consider a different situation where it does not matter whether one reverses both, then, of course, naloxone is the logical choice.

Baker   I would like to make an additional comment to what you brought out in terms of therapeutic effects in the case of biliary problems. We had an interesting experience recently with a patient, following liver transplantation, where there were biliary concretions that developed at the right and left biliary tracts; our radiologists were unable to instrument these concretions out of the biliary tree, so we gave a short course of infusion with glucagon which allowed the biliary tree to dilate sufficiently to let the concretions be pushed out by invasive radiology. A further comment that I would like to make in this line is that we really need a therapeutically applicable choleretic, which glucagon is not, one that we could give continuously for certain types of liver conditions. One would be cystic fibrosis, for example, with special relation to the kind of liver disease that occurs in cystic fibrosis where there are small biliary concretions that develop in the bile ducts and the liver; if we had a means to consistently keep the bile more liquid, this might provide an effective treatment or prevention for this type of liver condition.

Lefèbvre   If I may comment on that, I would like to say that maybe in this indication, Dr Baker, one could use glucagon. We diabetologists are used to treating diabetic patients for years using an insulin pump. They receive their insulin through a small portable pump, and I think that in patients with the type of disease that you are talking about, one could easily imagine using such a pump to deliver the very small doses of glucagon that would be required for the prolonged treatment of those critical chronic diseases.

Baker I think it is a very interesting idea and, since many of these patients are living increasingly to adulthood, it would be very useful to study this.

Vilardell To those conditions one might perhaps add sclerosing cholangitis, which I think would be a similar model where there often are bile plugs sitting on bile ducts and where, I imagine, that keeping bile fluid would probably help patients who are waiting for a transplant, for example ...

General Discussion

Oriol-Bosch   I would like to begin this general discussion by placing two basic questions relating to the physiology of glucagon. In the first place, is there any information about glucagon's secretory pattern? Is it known if glucagon is secreted in a more or less continuous fashion or if it belongs to the group of hormones that are secreted in a pulsatile manner? This is a very relevant question for the physiological understanding of its behaviour and also has very important pharmacological implications. The second question has to do with the existing information about the dynamics of the glucagon receptors, their turnover, replacement and generation. The physiological response may be conditioned not only by the actual levels of the hormone, but by its previous levels, which may have modified the receptor concentrations at the target cells.

Lefèbvre   Those are two very interesting questions. In the first place pulsa-tility. *In vitro* studies performed by Stagner and Samols (Stagner JI, Samols E, Weir GC. *J Clin Biol* 1980; 65:939–942) in Louisville, Kentucky, have shown that glucagon is secreted in a pulsatile manner which is also the case with insulin. This has been shown on isolated perfused canine pancreas and is completely independent of all the pharmacological effects that one can check; it is supposed to be due to some kind of intrapancreatic ganglionic pulsatile activity. *In vivo*, Goodner and his colleagues reported (Goodner CJ, Walike BC, Koerker DJ *et al. Science* 1977; 195:177–179) that in baboons and other monkeys, plasma glucagon levels were oscillating, that insulin was oscillating and that insulin and glucagon were oscillating out of phase, which I find extremely interesting. They also showed in the same monkeys that liver glucose output oscillates in synchrony with glucagon, which seems to indicate that these are really physiological mechanisms we are dealing with. Now concerning the effects of glucagon, if one infuses glucagon continuously either in dog or man one may see hyperglycaemia, for instance, due to an increased liver glucose output which will rise to a maximum and then go down again, despite the fact that you are still infusing glucagon. This is the so-called 'evanescent' effect of glucagon, which brings me to the second question. This has been attributed to some type of down-regulation of the receptor by glucagon, as has been shown for other hormones or, more basically, to some kind of desensitization of the receptor by the hormone. The intimate mechanism of the desensitization is not known exactly. It has been investigated but it is not known yet. Now dealing with the effect of glucagon on liver glucose output, there has been a beautiful study done in Seattle by Weigle (Weigle DS, Koerker DJ, Goodner CJ. *Am J Physiol* 1984; 247: E564–E568) on isolated perfused hepatocytes. A given amount of glucagon administered continuously to those hepatocytes produces a certain amount of glucose output. But when you give the same amount of glucagon intermittently, in a pulsatile manner, you get a greater glucose output than when it is given continuously. We have attempted to reproduce that in man (Palisso G, Scheen AJ, Luyckx AS *et al. Am J Physiol* 1987; 251: E1–E7) but have been unable to show that greater effect of pulsatile glucagon in man. Nonetheless, at the same time we were using somatostatin to inhibit endogenous secretion and a continuous insulin replacement, so what we are doing now is to give glucagon and insulin in a pulsatile out-of-phase manner to reproduce the physiological conditions, and we are very expectant as to what the results of this will be. Therefore, to summarize what I have said, glucagon is secreted in a pulsatile manner, at least *in vitro*, and intermittent glucagon at equivalent doses has a higher efficacy than continuously administered glucagon.

Oriol-Bosch Then it would seem that glucagon resembles other polypeptide hormones in the physiological behaviour of its secretory pattern and perhaps other similarities may also be expected to occur . . .

Carr-Locke Could you just clarify this pulsatility a little bit more? What order of timing are we talking about both in the naturally occurring situation and in the experiments?

Lefèbvre The natural cycles last between 12 and 18 min, that is the range. It is a little bit shorter for insulin, but as I said, they are out of phase. Anyhow, the glucagon cycles are around 14 min. The amplitude in the peripheral blood of man and monkeys is around $6\,pg\,ml^{-1}$, so you need a very sensitive assay to depict them and to make all the determinations, quadruplicate them removing all the noise and, of course, to use computer analyses of the measured data, because these are things that are not simply evident. You have to feed a computer and readjust the curves. Dr Carr-Locke, I think it would be very interesting to see in your studies if giving glucagon intermittently would magnify the measured effects. You would have to use the low doses you have been using, the lowest efficacious doses and give them in a pulsatile manner to see if this works. Is that what you were thinking about?

Carr-Locke Yes, that would be very nice. Of course, we are talking about the fasting state here, and it is interesting to see that this frequency may or may not be in time with the migration motor complex (MMC) of the bowel. Do you think there is a connection between that, or is it too much to expect?

Lefèbvre I am afraid this has not been studied for glucagon. Nobody has done this. There are only two groups in the world who have measured those pulsations, Goodner and his colleagues, as I already mentioned, and also for insulin someone nearer to you, Turner and his group in Oxford (Lang DA, Mathews DR, Peto PJ et al. N Engl J Med 1979; 301:1023–1027). But what you are suggesting has never been studied. There are many more data concerning insulin pulsatility. Mathews and his group attempted to modify the rhythm of the pulsations by all possible pharmacological means, those that you have also used (Mathews DR, Lang DA, Burnett MA et al. Diabetologia 1983; 24:231–237). But no one has been able to modify basically the rhythm for insulin. The only thing that you can modify is the amplitude. After a meal the amplitude is much greater, but the period remains the same (Hansen BC, Jen K-LC, Belbez-Pek S et al. J Clin Endocrinol Metab 1982; 54:785–792).

Nikolov Glucagon can stop motility of the smooth muscle from the oesophagus to the rectum, but is this a physiological or a pharmacological action?

Lefèbvre Yes, it is true that glucagon decreases the activity of the smooth muscle from the oesophagus to the rectum, but from what I have seen, read, and sometimes written, none of these effects have ever been reported as being physiological, with the exception of those found by Carr-Locke in the sphincter of Oddi and related structures (Carr-Locke DL, Gregg JA, Aoki TT. Dig Dis Sci 1983; 62:312–320). Most probably all the other effects are not physiologically relevant. I have never seen it reported that physiological doses of glucagon, which are ten or a hundred thousand times lower than what most radiologists or endoscopists have been using, could really affect the motility of the gut. Therefore, I believe that these are purely pharmacological effects.

Skucas Moving on to a different subject, Dr Maruyama, you discussed before the effect of anticholinergics in oesophageal hypotonia. It is my impression that the anticholinergics have a very small effect as far as inducing hypotonia of the oesophagus is concerned and that they only play a limited role in this aspect. Do you disagree with that?

Maruyama No. You are right, anticholinergics have very little effect on the relaxation of the oesophagus.

Skucas So why use them then?

Maruyama Because they are better than nothing.

Skucas I cannot argue with an answer like that!

Maruyama We must also remember the sedating effect, because anticholinergics give the patients some sedation, and what is also important, they produce a certain relaxation of the stomach, and in air-contrast examinations of the stomach, in order to get an optimal mucosal detail of the oesophagus, the stomach should also be relaxed to get a full distension not only of the oesophagus but of the stomach itself. This is the main reason why we use anticholinergics.

Nikolov Dr Skucas, what do you think about the intramuscular use of glucagon in children for safety reasons? Do you have any personal opinion on that?

Skucas As far as the relative merits of intravenous *versus* intramuscular glucagon, both in adults and children, to me they simply revolve around a question of cost. If I can use a much smaller dose of glucagon intravenously at a much lower cost, I will do so, that is the established practice, at least in the United States. As far as children are concerned and where the doses are lower, at least in my hospital they do receive the appropriate intramuscular dose of glucagon. First because the cost does not enter as much into consideration, and second because the veins are much more difficult to find, which makes the intramuscular injection much easier. So answering your question, in children we do use glucagon much more often intramuscularly.

Nikolov My next question is to Dr Maruyama. You have recommended the use of atropine even though you know that it gives patients great discomfort. What are the advantages of combining glucagon with atropine? Because I did not quite understand how you could restore completely the normal motility of the gastrointestinal system 20 min after using glucagon and then get no patient discomfort due to atropine ...

Maruyama To me, the most important thing is that glucagon does not inhibit gastric juice secretion, and that is the reason why I have to use atropine, in order to decrease gastric juice secretion.

Nikolov Is this your own opinion or is it shared, to your knowledge, by other practising radiologists?

Maruyama Well, of course, this is my experience, but the general consensus as far as I know is also that. Although glucagon does inhibit gastric acid secretion, it does not decrease or block the production of gastric juice.

Nikolov Does the presence of gastric juice in the stomach interfere significantly with your work and the quality of your films?

Maruyama Yes, it creates a serious problem when we are trying to obtain a very fine mucosal pattern in order to demonstrate these very subtle irregular mucosal erosions, specially in the proximal part of the lesion, when screening for cancer. Of course, atropine sulphate makes the patient very thirsty, which may be very discomforting, but nevertheless I would still recommend the use of atropine sulphate first if you want to obtain excellent mucosal details in double-contrast X-ray examinations of the stomach.

Lefèbvre I would like to ask David Carr-Locke about that new issue of infusing glucagon to help reduce jaundice pre-operatively. What is your basic idea? As I see it, to start with you have a patient with a mechanical obstruction to bile excretion and then by endoscopy you place a catheter or a prosthesis and resolve the obstruction and then, by giving glucagon, you increase the amount of bile coming through the catheter and in addition to that you may even get a more fluid bile. Is that it?

Carr-Locke Yes. Basically that is the principle. I have come around to it based on two different clinical experiences related to the same principle even if not from direct evidence. One is the fact that glucagon has been used in small children after operations for biliary atresia of which one of the complicating factors is the temporary blockage of the anastomosis leading to cholangitis, and there is a Japanese paper that suggests that using glucagon this may not happen (Watanabe Y, Todani T, Kobayashi T *et al. Z Kinderchir* 1983; 38:83–87). The other situation is percutaneous drainage of the bile ducts which is now less and less practised in fact. But the study using glucagon in that situation suggests that the degree and rate of bilirubin fall are greater with glucagon than with placebo. So based on that it seems sensible to apply it to the situation which is now very common, where we are relieving a mechanical problem, whether it is benign or malignant is irrelevant for the moment, in the bile duct temporarily, either by putting in an internal drainage prosthesis or an external catheter, as I have already shown. The problem we all have is that we do not know how long to wait between doing this and operating. There are a number of factors that we measure but the shorter that time, of course, the better for the patient. If we could reduce the level of jaundice and some other factors that are excreted in the bile, that have not been excreted in the obstructed state, and if glucagon may achieve that, it would be an advantage. But really it is only speculation at the moment.

Lefèbvre There is another question I would like to add. To what extent is bile flow dependent upon splanchnic blood flow? When splanchnic blood flow increases, is bile flow increased automatically?

Carr-Locke   There is a relationship, and glucagon as you know increases blood flow in certain experimental animals at the same time as it is a choleretic.

Lefèbvre   Yes indeed. The effect of glucagon on splanchnic blood flow has been known for 20 years. Actually, in 1964 I published a paper on that in the dog (Lefèbvre PJ, Beaujeau M. *Arch Int Physiol Biochem* 1964; 72:9–16), and I think that Professor Vilardell has just had new information about those effects recently.

Vilardell   Yes, I recently heard a paper by a group of hepatologists led by Lebrec (Lee SS, Moreau R, Hadengue A *et al*. *Gastroenterol Clin Biol* 1987; 11:160A) who have done the original work on propanolol decreasing portal pressure and he has shown conclusively in man an increase in splanchnic blood flow due to glucagon very clearly, particularly in cirrhotic patients. I wonder if this will have any further application, but surely that may have something to do with blood flow through the liver, and certainly bile flow later on, so indeed, there may be a connection. A comment I have for Dr Carr-Locke is that, in fact, many of these patients in whom you are going to do bile drainage may be getting a sump, or may already have white bile for instance, or bile which has very different properties from normal bile, so it would be interesting to study the composition of bile during glucagon infusion in that sort of patient because it may prove to be quite different from normal. Some show very dark bile and others have a whitish bile ...

Baker   It seems to me that a simple way to think about it would be that anything that increases canalicular bile flow is likely to increase the flow of anything that will pass into the bile, that is to say, anything that is water-soluble and that is able to pass into the bile out of the canaliculus. Of course, conjugated bilirubin would be one of those along with many other substances. It seems to me that you might expect perhaps less of the choleretic effect but mainly an increase in water, which is what we would think glucagon might do on soluble fat substances such as cholesterol for example. So there might be less of an effect on cholesterol excretion into bile.

Carr-Locke   I hate to complicate the issue, but I do not think it is quite as straightforward as that, and the reason I am saying this is because if you look at the radiological aspects of this phenomenon that I reported earlier, glucagon has been shown to enhance iotroxamide excretion, while other studies using different contrast agents have shown quite different results, and yet they all have potentially the same kind of fat and water solubility in bile, but still glucagon can affect them quite differently, and we really do not understand why that is. Iotroxamide is obviously one of the more favourably influenced ones, but there are some other ones that do not seem to change at all. So quite what the relationship is between the effect of glucagon and the excretion of other anions I think we just do not know yet.

Baker   I am not particularly familiar with iotroxamide, but are all those contrast agents conjugated to a certain degree to water-soluble compounds?

Carr-Locke   Yes. To some extent they are all rendered more water soluble by a conjugation process, but whether this happens to the same degree for all of them I do not think we know for most of them.

Lefèbvre   Going back to your paper Dr Carr-Locke, I am very interested in putting your findings into a physiological perspective because I think the effects that you have shown are actually seen with doses which are within physiological levels. Therefore, if you take a pure glucose meal, 100 g glucose in 400 ml of water and you drink it, you will see glucagon decrease, but what happens to the Oddi sphincter then? Also in the opposite situation where you would take a mixed meal containing proteins, you would see a rise in glucagon. I wonder if after this mixed meal what you observe in terms of mechanics there is consistent with the rise of glucagon ...

Carr-Locke   The problem of course is that we are limited by the techniques that we use to measure these things, which is the reason for not being able to do them in the fed state. What I mean is that it would be very interesting to know the effect of certain foodstuffs, to take the physiology a further step back without actually giving the hormone exogenously, which, of course, is artificial. But it really is quite impossible to do that. One way around the problem is to infuse a liquid meal of some sort into the duodenum, which again is not really a terribly physiological thing to do, but it has been done for fat, and in that case you can measure the response of the sphincter of Oddi. I cannot answer that specific question of the effect of a mixed meal, but that is what we are trying to reproduce by infusing the exogenous peptide.

Lefèbvre   From a pathophysiological point of view, during the digestion of a meal, what you would expect would be the relaxation of the sphincter of Oddi because bile should come there to help digestion. My point is that with a mixed meal you do have an increase in glucagon, and in addition to its effects, maybe those small increases in secretin levels may contribute to produce that relaxation.

Carr-Locke   Indeed. But one must not forget that this effect is only one effect of many, as for instance the effect of CCK, which will be released by the mixed meal and which may far outweigh the effect of glucagon or summate with it. Again we are back to the point where we do not know the effect of the two peptides working simultaneously.

Lefèbvre   What is the effect of CCK on the sphincter of Oddi?

Carr-Locke   It is again a relaxing effect.

Vilardell   What about the chronic pancreatitis? Has anyone studied patients with sclerosing pancreatitis where you may have low glucagon levels?

Carr-Locke The only studies I know of with glucagon and pressure studies in chronic pancreatitis are Japanese (Okazaki K, Yamamoto Y, Ito K. *Gastroenterology* 1986; 91:409–418), looking at the pancreatic duct pressure changes, not so much at the sphincter changes, because in fact, sphincter of Oddi dynamics do not seem to be terribly different. The only reservation is that the alcoholic patients are different, but that is another topic. In terms of pancreatic duct pressure changes I think the literature is a little bit confused because some of the more recent work is very difficult to understand, with very high pressures being shown in the pancreatic duct of patients with chronic pancreatitis which I am not sure about. But glucagon does seem to reduce those because of its anti-secretory effects on pancreatic juice flow.

Nikolov One fact that I find disturbing in general is the extreme confusion that is created when investigating glucagon, for instance by factors such as species variations, extrapolation to humans and discrimination between physiological and pharmacological effects of the studies, because without standardizations what we get is different results and no satisfactory answers.

Lefèbvre The only comment that I can make is that animal studies can only be applied to humans if properly investigated in humans, and that in the field of glucagon I think that since we are dealing with a safe physiological compound, as soon as it is ethical to do a study in man, one should try to see if it has an effect in man, because that is the only sound way to come quickly to meaningful answers.

Vilardell Has anyone been able to study patients with glucagonoma in relation to any of the physiological effects of glucagon?

Lefèbvre Oh yes, there are several studies, some done by us, in which the main features of glucagonoma are a very mild diabetes, an extreme perturbation in the circulating levels of amino-acids, and a very peculiar dermatitis, and even though this is a field that has not been touched at all today, it might be worth discussing it in a future meeting such as this one.

Vilardell Well, I think that this brings to an end our first session of general discussion, but before we adjourn, I think that we should give Professor Lefèbvre, who will not be attending the rest of the meeting, a last opportunity to speak before he leaves.

Oriol-Bosch Yes. Unfortunately Professor Lefèbvre is unable to stay to the end due to other unavoidable commitments. This is the reason why we have decided to split the General Discussion of this meeting into two sessions, morning and afternoon, in order to be able to have his very valuable contribution at least in one of these, so Professor Lefèbvre we would appreciate very much if it is you who closes this morning session for us.

Lefèbvre   Thank you. First of all I would like to say that I must apologize for being unable to stay with you, and very specially to all the colleagues that I will not be listening to, although certainly I will read their manuscripts with great expectation, because the whole subject of the effects of glucagon is really crucial. There has been an immense load of literature on the basic concepts involved in liver regeneration but, meanwhile, in all our hospitals we know every month or every two months of a young patient who dies from acute liver insufficiency, and I think that the approach of giving glucagon with insulin and those extremely interesting data Professor Fehér will present, and that I know of, and those that our Japanese colleagues will present, are extremely important and therefore I think that this will be a great contribution which again, I am sorry to miss. It has been a pleasure to be here and let us hope that this will not be the last get together of this kind, which I find very enriching. Thank you.

Hepatology Session

7
Experimental evidence of the hepatotrophic effect of insulin and glucagon

K. FUJIWARA, I. OGATA, S. MISHIRO, Y. OHTA, Y. OKA,
K. TAKATSUKI, Y. SATO, S. HAYASHI, S. YAMADA and H. OKA

INTRODUCTION

Insulin and glucagon have been reported to be hepatotrophic since they are effective in potentiating liver regeneration and protecting the liver from atrophy[1-7]. These results were obtained under experimental conditions with a deficiency of endogenous insulin and glucagon induced by portal deprivation[1,2,4], evisceration[5,6], or alloxan diabetes[3,7]. Thus, it is possible that the effect was only supplementary to the restoration from retardation. Both hormones have been applied to the treatment of acute hepatic failure[8-11]. The action, however, seems to be complicated. The favourable effect of glucagon and insulin on the survival of mice with fulminant viral hepatitis reported by Farivar et al.[8] might be the result of hepatoprotection, since 24 h after viral infection they observed morphologically an attenuation of hepatocellular necrosis with the therapy. The promotion of liver functions besides the stimulation of liver regeneration could explain the rapid improvement of prothrombin time and total bilirubin levels after hormone infusion in alcoholic hepatitis patients reported by Baker et al.[9].

This situation prompted us to investigate whether insulin and glucagon stimulate liver regeneration under conditions with intact secretion of endogenous hormones and whether they have additional effects when used for liver damage. We also evaluated the efficacy of both hormones in the treatment of acute hepatic failure.

STIMULATION OF LIVER REGENERATION BY GLUCAGON AND INSULIN UNDER INTACT SECRETION OF ENDOGENOUS HORMONES

Male Wistar rats underwent 67% partial hepatectomy and received a sub-cutaneous injection of $40 \, mU \, kg^{-1}$ insulin and/or $25 \, \mu g \, kg^{-1}$ glucagon solution every 2 h along with an intraperitoneal injection of 5 μCi of [^{3}H]thymidine (^{3}H-TdR) after 12 h and until 2 h before sacrifice. Wedge biopsy of the liver (about 0.05 g removal) was performed in these rats three times at 20, 30 and 40 h, or at 30, 40 and 50 h. They were sacrificed 10 h after the last biopsy and the liver was excised. With these liver specimens, ^{3}H-TdR incorporation into DNA was determined. The values at varying times were plotted serially, and a profile of the incorporation curve was made for each rat to find the times the values were assumed to reach a maximum (Tm). Each rat was classified in one of four groups according to Tm defined as shown in Figure 7.1.

The results are shown in Table 7.1. Of 20 control rats, 14 showed a Tm longer than 51 h. In contrast, there were only five in the same group out of 20 rats treated with glucagon and insulin; a greater number of rats were found to have a Tm shorter than 50 h. The difference from the control rats was significant. In rats treated with either insulin or glucagon alone, 50% showed a Tm between 30 and 50 h.

These results may indicate that the first burst of DNA synthesis after partial hepatectomy reached a maximum sooner in the glucagon and insulin treated rats than in the control rats. ^{3}H-TdR incorporation into DNA was increased in all groups. Therefore, it can be assumed that both hormones increased the number of hepatocytes entering the G1-phase of the cell cycle, suggesting that both hormones acted on the early G1-phase. We conclude from this experiment that both hormones stimulate liver cell proliferation under intact secretion of endogenous insulin and glucagon. Recently comparable results were reported by De Diego et al.[13]

PROMOTION OF RESTORATION OF LIVER FUNCTION BY GLUCAGON AND INSULIN IN LIVER INJURY

When rats were given an intraperitoneal injection of $40 \, mg \, kg^{-1}$ of di-methylnitrosamine (DMN), SGPT values reached a maximum within 36 h and attained a plateau within 8 h. Some rats died thereafter but, in the survivors, the values decreased after 3 days. These rats were simultaneously injected

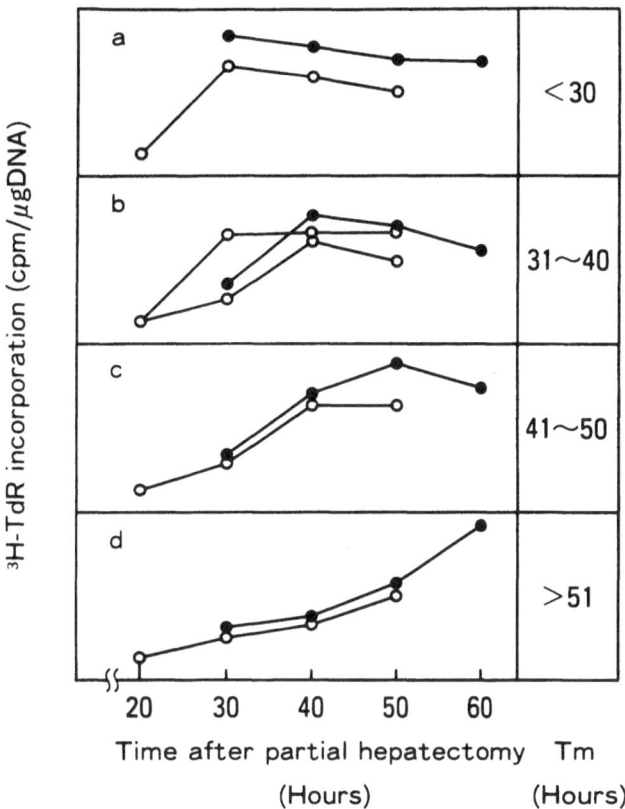

Figure 7.1 Patterns of cumulative ³H-TdR incorporation into DNA of post-hepatectomized rat liver, and times at which the incorporation value reaches a maximum (Tm). Open circles indicate data from the experiments where rats underwent hepatic wedge biopsy at 20, 30 and 40 h, and were sacrificed at 50 h after partial hepatectomy. Closed circles indicate data from the experimental rats undergoing biopsy at 30, 40 and 50 h and sacrificed at 60 h. (Takatsuki K et al.[12])

with 75 μg kg^{-1} glucagon and 120 mU kg^{-1} insulin subcutaneously six times at 4 h intervals immediately or 24 h after giving DMN. They were sacrificed at the indicated times with an intraperitoneal injection of 20 μCi of ³H-TdR before 1 h and liver function tests and hepatic DNA synthesis were determined.

As shown in Table 7.2, when hormone (GI) treatment was started immediately after giving DMN, hepatic DNA synthesis tended to increase at 24 h compared to the control rats, though SGPT and prothrombin time (PT) did not change. In the case of GI treatment starting 24 h after giving DMN, however, DNA synthesis and PT in the control group were significantly lower at 72 h than at 48 h. This may imply that stimulation of hepatocyte proliferation in

Table 7.1 Effect of glucagon and/or insulin on the time (Tm) of maximum ^{3}H-TdR incorporation into post-hepatectomized rat liver DNA

| Treatment | Groups* | | | | | Multiple |
	a	b	c	d	Total	comparison
Control	0	2	4	14	20	
Insulin	0	4	4	9	17	
Glucagon	0	3	3	6	12	
Insulin + glucagon	2	6	7	5	20	$p = 0.303$ vs control

Figures indicate number of rats. *Groups a, b, c and d according to Tm are defined in Figure 7.1. Kruskal-Wallis test between control and treated rats: $\chi_0^2[3] = 9.028$, $p = 0.028$ (Takatsuki K et al.[12])

Table 7.2 Effect of hormone (GI) treatment on SGPT, prothrombin time (PT) and hepatic DNA synthesis in rats given a single dose of dimethylnitrosamine (DMN)

Groups	No. of rats	SGPT (Karmen Unit)	PT (s)	DNA synthesis (cpm (mgDNA)$^{-1}$)
GI treatment immediately after giving DMN				
At 24 h[a]:				
Control	9	730 ± 420	26.8 ± 8.0	297 ± 100[b]
GI-treated	9	590 ± 230	25.7 ± 7.0	416 ± 141**
GI treatment 24 h after giving DMN				
At 48 h:				
Control	9	545 ± 240	20.9 ± 2.7	535 ± 133
GI-treated	8	570 ± 390	20.4 ± 2.4	492 ± 120
At 72 h:				
Control	8	390 ± 160	16.7 ± 2.5*	328 ± 156*
GI-treated	8	320 ± 160	18.0 ± 3.1	305 ± 186

[a] hours after giving DMN. [b] Values are the mean ± SD in surviving rats. *$p < 0.01$ vs 48 h, and **$p < 0.1$ vs control group (Student's t-test)

the presence of these hormones occurred within 24 h, but not thereafter, though the reason for this remains obscure.

In order to find any effect other than the stimulation of cell proliferation in the recovery phase from liver injury, GI treatment was started with this model after 24 h and continued for 3 days, and hepatic protein content was determined serially at Days 5, 7 and 9. The protein content would provide a good parameter for the extent of liver damage, especially in this model where injury was the result of inhibited protein synthesis. Table 7.3 shows the results obtained with this model. On Day 5, hepatic protein content was significantly lower in the control and hormone-treated groups than in normal rats. On Day 9 it was observed that although this reduction persisted in the control group, the content increased and normalized. Nor did concomitantly measured hepatic DNA content differ between the two groups until Day 9. Body and liver

Table 7.3 Hepatic protein and DNA contents and body weight in rats with 3 days of GI treatment starting 24 h after a single dose of dimethylnitrosamine (means ± SD in surviving rats, n in parentheses)

Groups	Day 5[a]	Day 7	Day 9
Total liver protein content (g)			
Control	$1.43 \pm 0.38^{\dagger\dagger}$ (7)	1.29 ± 0.26 (10)	$1.67 \pm 0.22^{\dagger\dagger}$ (9)
GI-treated	$1.60 \pm 0.25^{\dagger\dagger}$ (7)	$1.56 \pm 0.33^{*}$ (10)	$2.17 \pm 0.57^{**}$ (9)
Normal	2.18 ± 0.27 (5)		2.29 ± 0.12 (5)
Total liver DNA content (mg)			
Control	$42.1 \pm 5.1^{\dagger\dagger}$ (7)	31.6 ± 5.9 (10)	$36.2 \pm 4.5^{\dagger}$ (9)
GI-treated	$39.1 \pm 6.3^{\dagger\dagger}$ (7)	33.4 ± 5.3 (10)	35.7 ± 8.1 (9)
Normal	25.3 ± 5.0 (5)		30.3 ± 1.9 (5)
Body weight (g)			
Control	230 ± 22 (7)	216 ± 23 (10)	$250 \pm 21^{\dagger\dagger}$ (9)
GI-treated	217 ± 23 (7)	225 ± 28 (10)	$243 \pm 26^{\dagger\dagger}$ (9)
Normal	234 ± 26 (5)		266 ± 11 (5)

[a] Days after giving DMN.
$p < :^{*}0.1$; $^{**}0.05$ *vs* control group and $p < :^{\dagger}0.05$; $^{\dagger\dagger}0.01$ *vs* normal group (Student's *t*-test)

weights were not different between the two groups. Therefore, this result may indicate the promotion of restoration of hepatocyte function by both hormones, probably by acting on injured and/or regenerating hepatocytes. This effect took some time to appear, as the normalization occurred 5 days after discontinuation of treatment. Such an effect must be considered besides the stimulation of hepatocyte proliferation in the evaluation of glucagon and insulin for treatment of acute hepatic failure. The hepatoprotective effect was not observed with this model, as is seen by the changes in SGPT and PT values.

EFFECTIVENESS OF GLUCAGON AND INSULIN IN THE TREATMENT OF HEPATIC FAILURE

To evaluate the efficacy of GI treatment in hepatic failure, we used a DMN-induced model, since there is the excluding possibility that the effectiveness in fulminant murine hepatitis reported by Farivar et al.[8] might also be caused by its protective action against murine viral attack, and the hepatotoxic mechanism induced by DMN is quite different. In the preliminary experiments we studied the effect of GI treatment on survival using rats with a single dose of DMN as well as of D-galactosamine or carbon tetrachloride, but did not succeed in proving its effectiveness. The possibilities were that rats given a fatal dosage of hepatotoxins would not survive even if they had been effectively treated or that the efficacy would be limited to a certain degree of severity. Therefore, we employed a progressive injury.

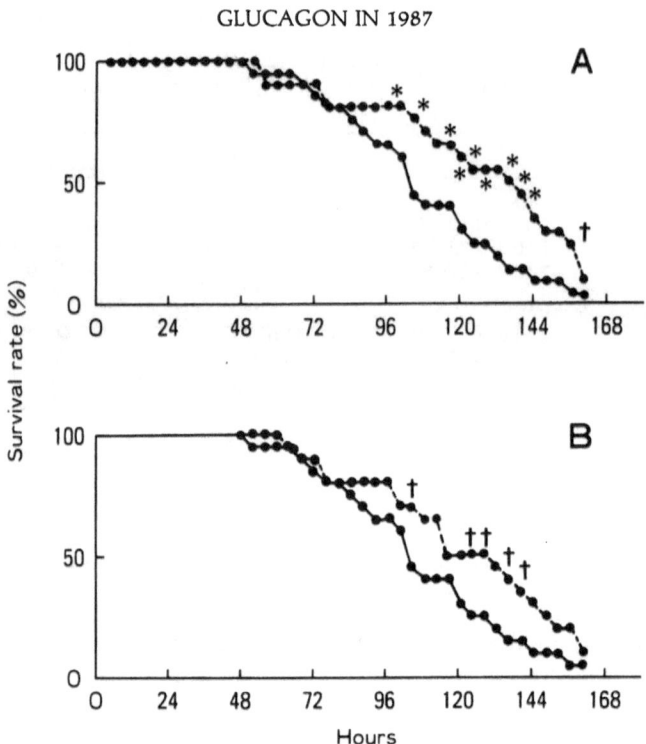

Figure 7.2 Effect of GI treatment starting at 24 h on survival rate of rats with successive administration of dimethylnitrosamine. Open circles indicate survival rate in the GI-treated group and closed circles indicate the survival rate in the control group. Panel A: results of 75 μg kg^{-1} glucagon and 120 mU kg^{-1} insulin; panel B: results of 7.5 μg kg^{-1} glucagon and 120 mU kg^{-1} insulin. *$p < 0.05$, †$p < 0.1$ vs control group (Cutler-Ederer's test)

Rats received an intraperitoneal injection of 15 mg kg^{-1} DMN every 24 h until death. After the first 24 h they were given GI treatment at varying doses of glucagon and insulin, similarly until death. Figure 7.2 shows the survival of these rats when treated with a combination of 75 or 7.5 μg kg^{-1} glucagon and 120 mU kg^{-1} insulin. In the case of 75 μg kg^{-1} glucagon and 120 mU kg^{-1} insulin, the survival rate was significantly enhanced by treatment after 100 h, but this enhancement disappeared after 140 h. When the glucagon dose was reduced to one tenth of that dose the enhancement was less evident. A similar degree of effectiveness was also found when the insulin dose was reduced to one half of the previous dose. However, higher doses of glucagon and insulin or both hormones alone did not affect the survival rate (Table 7.4). The optimal glucagon dose (0.45 mg kg^{-1} d^{-1}) is almost comparable with that reported by Farivar et al.[8], although the insulin dose in that study was much smaller.

In another experiment, surviving rats treated with 75 μg kg^{-1} glucagon and 120 mU kg^{-1} insulin were sacrificed at 100 or 120 h, and liver function tests

Table 7.4 Effect of GI treatment at varying doses of glucagon and insulin on the survival rate of rats with successive administration of dimethylnitrosamine

| | | Glucagon (μg kg^{-1} (4 h)$^{-1}$) | | | | | | |
		0	7.5	15	37.5	75	150	300
Insulin	0					−		
(mU kg^{-1} (4 h)$^{-1}$)	60					+		
	120	−	+	+	+	+	−	−
						+ +		
	240					−		

Effect of GI treatment on survival rate is evaluated by Cutler-Ederer's test: − = unchanged ($p > 0.1$); + = improved ($p < 0.1$); + + = significantly improved ($p < 0.05$); between 100 and 140 h compared to control group

Table 7.5 Effect of GI treatment on prothrombin time (PT), serum albumin (SA) and blood glucose (BG) levels in surviving rats with successive dimethylnitrosamine administration (values are means ± SD)

Groups	No. of rats	PT (s)	SA (g dl^{-1})	BG (mg dl^{-1})
Survivors at 100 h:				
Control	13	18.1 ± 3.3	2.28 ± 0.27	92 ± 24
GI-treated	19	19.2 ± 4.6	2.31 ± 0.32	93 ± 23
Survivors at 120 h:				
Control	7	28.7 ± 3.2	2.00 ± 0.32	88 ± 18
GI-treated	13	25.2 ± 2.9*	2.24 ± 0.20	108 ± 18*
			*	
Normal	5	11.2 ± 0.6	3.20 ± 0.15	117 ± 10

*$p < 0.05$ vs control group (Student's *t*-test)

and blood glucose levels were determined. Table 7.5 shows these results. At 100 h when the enhanced survival rate by GI treatment started to appear, there was no difference in PT or serum albumin levels between the hormone treated and control groups. However, at 120 h, when liver injury progressed further and the enhancement of the survival rate became prominent, the deranged values of these parameters were significantly attenuated by hormone treatment. Blood glucose at 100 h was decreased in both groups, but levels returned to normal at 120 h in the hormone treated group. The hypoglycaemia caused by this treatment in humans[9] was not found in this experiment. A beneficial effect of both hormones on liver injury was strongly suggested. The improvement of the survival rate would be such a result, since the cause of death can be assumed to be due to hepatic failure, as is seen in our preliminary experiment where survival time in rats given a single dose of DMN is negatively correlated with PT measured at 24 h.

SUMMARY AND CONCLUSIONS

In these experiments we found in the first place that glucagon and insulin accelerated DNA synthesis in post-hepatectomized regenerating liver of normal rats. Secondly, both hormones promoted restoration of liver protein contents in DMN-intoxicated rats and, finally, survival rate was enhanced by hormone treatment along with an attenuation of deranged serum albumin levels and PT in rats with DMN-induced progressive liver injury.

We conclude that glucagon and insulin may be hepatotrophic and beneficial for the treatment of liver injury.

References

1. Starzl TE, Francavilla A, Halgrimson CG, Francavilla FR, Porter KA, Brown TH, Putnam CW. The origin, hormonal nature, and action of hepatotrophic substances in portal venous blood. *Surg Gynecol Obstet* 1973; 137: 179–199.
2. Starzl TE, Porter KA, Putnam CW. Intraportal insulin protects from the liver injury of portacaval shunt in dogs. *Lancet* 1975; 2: 1241–1242.
3. Starzl TE, Porter KA, Kashiwagi N, Lee IY, Russell WJI, Putnam CW. The effect of diabetes mellitus on portal blood hepatotrophic factors in dogs. *Surg Gynecol Obstet* 1977; 140: 549–562.
4. Starzl TE, Porter KA, Watanabe K, Putnam CW. Effects of insulin, glucagon, and insulin/glucagon infusions on liver morphology and cell division after complete portacaval shunt in dogs. *Lancet* 1976; 1: 821–825.
5. Bucher NLR, Swaffield MN. Regulation of hepatic regeneration in rats by synergistic action in insulin and glucagon. *Proc Natl Acad Sci USA* 1975; 72: 1157–1160.
6. Whittemore AD, Kasuya M, Voorhees AB Jr, Price JB Jr, Hepatic regeneration in the absence of portal viscera. *Surgery* 1975; 77: 419–426.
7. Barra R, Hall JC. Liver regeneration in normal and alloxan-induced diabetic rats. *J Exp Zool* 1977; 201: 93–100.
8. Farivar M, Wands JR, Isselbacher KJ, Bucher NLR. Effect of insulin and glucagon on fulminant murine hepatitis. *N Engl J Med* 1976; 295: 1517–1519.
9. Baker AL, Jaspan JB, Haines NW, Hatfield GE, Krager PS, Schneider JF. A randomized clinical trial of insulin and glucagon for treatment of alcoholic hepatitis: Progress report in 50 patients. *Gastroenterology* 1981; 80: 1410–1414.
10. Okita K, Matsuda S, Hata K, Morimoto T, Sasaki M, Fukumoto Y, Kodama T, Takemoto T. Clinical use of glucagon and insulin in therapy of fulminant hepatic failure. *Gastroenterol Jpn* 1979; 14; 453–457.
11. Oka H, Okita K, Fujiwara K. Glucagon and insulin therapy in fulminant hepatic failure in Japan. In: Picazo J, ed. *Glucagon in Gastroenterology and Hepatology.* Lancaster, Boston, The Hague: MTP Press, 1982: 171–180.
12. Takatsuki K, Fujiwara K, Hayashi S, Ota Y, Torii M, Mishiro S, Ogata I, Sakuma A, Oka H, Oda T. Acceleration of DNA synthesis in post-hepatectomized regenerating liver of normal rat by insulin and glucagon. *Life Sci* 1981; 29: 2609–2615.
13. De Diego JA, Molina LM, Buján J, Simón P, Gea M, Menchero A, Balibrea JL. Influence of the conjoint administration of insulin and glucagon upon hepatic regeneration. *Surg Gynecol Obstet* 1986; 163: 443–447.

DISCUSSION

Nikolov   Since I am interested myself in studying liver regeneration experimentally in *in vivo* models, I would like to know what technique you have utilized to perform subtotal hepatectomy in your rat model.

Fujiwara   I just performed partial hepatectomy according to Higgins and Anderson (Higgins GM, Anderson RM. *Arch Pathol* 1931; 12: 186–202).

Nikolov   Then, a second point I would raise is that there are many growth factors influencing the liver, and not just insulin and glucagon. Perhaps fibroblast growth factor and thrombocyte growth factor are also involved, so I would like to know if you have done any experimental work with factors other than glucagon and insulin.

Fujiwara   I have presented here my experience up to date, but certainly I would like to study other trophic factors, epidermal growth factor, for instance, which perhaps might lead to more effective models of therapy.

Nikolov   Why use the two factors together and not alone? Why do you not use just insulin, for instance?.

Fujiwara   As a matter of fact, we already have done this, as I mentioned before, in our initial experiments. In our model we tested glucagon and insulin alone, and then the combination of the two, and we found that the combination had a maximal trophic effect.

Baker   I think that having glucagon and insulin as the controls and being able to show that they had no effect is very important for the control of these studies.

Oka   I could add to this that we used glucagon and insulin because we have no other peptide hormones available for clinical use at the moment; EGF, fibroblast growth factor and other possible hepatotraphic factors are not yet available for clinical treatment, so we studied those that we knew could be applied to therapy currently. On the other hand, the hepatotrophic action of insulin is already established, since many experimental studies *in vivo* and *in vitro* have shown that insulin stimulates hepatic cell proliferation, but we do not have any conclusive data of the action of glucagon on hepatic regeneration except for that of Nancy Bucher's experiments in rats using eviscerated animals (Bucher NLR, Swaffield MN. *Proc Natl Acad Sci USA* 1975; 72: 1157–1160) and Leffert's studies (Leffert HL. *J Cell Biol* 1974; 62: 792–801), but no studies in humans.

Baker   I want to ask you about your current thoughts as to the relatively small differences that you have shown. Have you been able to do anything to enhance these differences in either DNA synthesis or survival, for example? Have you been able to pre-treat the animals in any way to enhance the differences, or have you found that if you give the insulin and glucagon before the dimethylnitrosamine you get a different effect? Have you had a chance to do those experiments?

Fujiwara We did actually perform another study where insulin/glucagon infusion was started immediately after a single injection of dimethyl-nitrosamine, and here we found an adverse effect. The reason, of course, is that insulin and glucagon enhance cytochrome P450 activation, leading to the production of metabolites such as hepatotoxin, so we changed the protocol.

Baker So you would probably get a similar result, I suppose, if you pretreated the animals with glucagon and insulin before you gave the di-methylnitrosamine?

Fukiwara Well, if we want to get a better improvement with this treatment we must change the model of hepatic injury, I mean we need a different hepatotoxin, like virus infection for instance.

Baker Let me ask you one more question. In your experiments, did you monitor blood sugar levels and, if so, what did you find?

Fujiwara In our last experiment we checked blood glucose levels and we got a result at 100 h, blood glucose was reduced below normal levels in both groups at 140 h. This reduction progressed, but insulin and glucagon infusion attenuated this reduction.

Baker I would like to ask just one more question on this general line. You said that in your insulin plus glucagon-treated group there were no differences in the liver weights in relation to the controls, did I understand that correctly?.

Fujiwara Yes, that is right, there were no differences.

Baker No difference? Does that bother you in terms of attributing this effect to hepatic regeneration rather than to some other metabolic effect, or is your conclusion that this is a metabolic effect on the liver, rather than regeneration *per se*?

Fujiwara I think liver weight is not related to the result of liver regeneration in the models we have employed here.

Baker But would you not expect a bigger liver in the treated animals if regeneration is actually the effect that your treatment is having?

Fujiwara No. You see, in hepatotoxin-induced models of liver injury, we usually get an enhancement of the liver weight in general, depending on the extent of the liver injury.

Oka I think that in the damaged liver the weight depends on the amount of fat and other things, so the weight of the liver is not quite that different from that of the regenerating liver. Therefore, insulin and glucagon do not increase liver weight.

Baker So, in terms of total DNA content or total protein content, you did see an increase in total protein content, but not in liver weight, did you not?

Fujiwara   Yes, that is right.

Nikolov   Were your rats immobilized during treatment? Because I think that would be a stress factor.

Fujiwara   No, they were not. The hormones were given subcutaneously and not via catheterization of the femoral vein.

8
Insulin and glucagon infusion therapy in acute alcoholic hepatitis

J. FEHÉR, A. CORNIDES, A. GÓGL, A. ROMÁNY, M. KÁRTESZI,
L. SZALAY and J. PICAZO

INTRODUCTION

Alcohol consumption is probably the commonest self-induced injury to the liver nowadays, and the most frequent cause of chronic liver disease. In Western countries the incidence of liver cirrhosis can be directly related to the quantity of consumed alcohol. The death rate in different communities correlates quite well with alcohol consumption[1]. Table 8.1 shows alcohol consumption (absolute alcohol in litres) in 1983, according to data from the World Health Organization. However, these data vary and, for instance, in the last ten years the consumption of alcohol *per capita* has decreased in France and increased in Hungary.

During the last 15 years alcoholic liver disease has increased markedly among women[2,3]. The susceptibility of women to alcoholic liver disease is much higher than it is for men. The 'safe' daily consumption is uncertain, but it can be considered that 50–60 g in men and 20–25 g in women may be an adequate figure. Alcoholic patients with cirrhosis have usually consumed about 190 g of alcohol daily for 10 years, although there are wide individual variations. In patients studied by us we found that 33% of those with chronic liver disease were alcoholic, while only 3.2% of the control patients could be defined as heavy drinkers[2].

Not everyone who drinks excessively develops liver damage. In a group of 526 unselected male alcoholics receiving treatment, liver function tests

Table 8.1   Alcohol consumption per year in some European countries

Country	Per capita *alcohol consumption per year* (L of absolute alcohol)
Portugal	13.5
France	13.1
Spain	12.8
Italy	12.3
Hungary	11.3
Switzerland	11.2
West Germany	11.0
East Germany	10.4
Austria	10.2

showed severe liver damage in a quarter of the cases, and milder liver damage in half of them. The numerous chronic alcoholics with completely normal liver pose an interesting problem. An explanation for this might be that there are genetic influences determining hepatic susceptibility to alcohol[1].

According to its clinical features, we divide alcoholic liver disease into four groups: fatty liver, alcoholic hepatitis, liver cirrhosis, and hepatocellular carcinoma. These diseases frequently overlap each other[4-6].

Alcoholic hepatitis usually appears as severe hepatic decompensation after particularly heavy drinking, perhaps precipitated by vomiting, diarrhoea, an acute infection or prolonged anorexia[1]. The patient is pyrexial and jaundiced. The liver is enlarged and tender, and an arterial bruit may be heard over it. The spleen is often impalpable. Ascites may develop rapidly. Faeces are usually pale. Biochemical tests show raised serum alkaline phosphatase and transaminase activities, as well as hyperbilirubinaemia, hypo-albuminaemia, hypergammaglobulinaemia. The morphologic picture of the liver is characteristic, and the prognosis is bad. Immunologically it is characterized by polyclonal hypergammaglobulinaemia, elevated IgA plasma concentration and IgA deposits in the hepatic sinusoids. Acute alcoholic hepatitis is very often fatal.

The established treatment of acute alcoholic hepatitis is mainly supportive and should include *abstinence*, *bed* rest and high *calorie* intake, the so-called ABC of management. However, there is no generally accepted specific treatment for the illness. Several controlled clinical trials of corticosteroid therapy have been performed in patients with alcoholic hepatitis, but these do not provide unequivocal evidence of benefit[7,8]. The effects of other drugs (colchicine, silibinin, D-penicillamine) require more detailed examination[9-11] before they can be prescribed for the broad group of patients with alcoholic hepatitis.

'On the basis of animal experimental studies[12] and the beneficial results of some clinical trials[13-15], we examined the effect of combined insulin and glucagon infusion therapy for the treatment of acute alcoholic hepatitis in a multicentre study.

MATERIALS AND METHODS

Sixty-six patients with acute alcoholic hepatitis were selected for study in a multicentre trial. Those with odd numbers (1, 3, 5, etc.) had infusions with insulin and glucagon; those with even numbers (2, 4, 6, etc.) served as controls with placebo treatment (single blind trial). All the patients in the study agreed to participate giving fully informed consent to a protocol according to the Declaration of Helsinki. Patients were kept on a 2200 calorie diet and were given nutritional supplement when caloric intake seemed inadequate. Abstinence from ethanol was carefully advised. Patients were treated with protein restriction, oral antibiotics for bowel sterilization, bowel wash, liquid antacids, vitamins, lactulose, free-radical scavengers, and fresh blood transfusions, as and whenever necessary. Vital functions were monitored and electrolyte disturbances, if present, were promptly corrected. Patients with severe gastrointestinal bleeding, pancreatitis, and those who refused treatment after detailed information were excluded from the trial.

The diagnosis was based on clinical, biochemical and morphological data. Liver biopsy was not performed in 15 of the cases because the prothrombin time was below 50% of the normal value.

The clinical parameters for diagnosis were age, duration and quantity of alcohol consumption, hepatomegaly and splenomegaly, as measured in cm below the costal margin. The biochemical parameters were aspartate aminotransferase (AST), alanine aminotransferase (ALT), γ-glutamyltranspeptidase (GGT), total bilirubin, γ-globulin, and prothrombin time.

The histological alteration of liver biopsy material was studied in 51 cases (26 patients from the control and 25 from the treatment group). Liver biopsies were performed subcutaneously with a Menghini needle and tissue was fixed in 4% formalin. Sections were stained with haematoxylin–eosin for reticulin and by Masson's trichrome stain. The histological examination of all tissue sections was done by two pathologists without prior knowledge of clinical and laboratory data, nor whether patients belonged to the control or the treatment groups. Besides acute inflammatory reactions, previous alterations of liver steatosis, portal fibrosis and cirrhosis were analysed.

Patients in the treatment group received an infusion of 10 U insulin and 1 mg glucagon in 500 ml of 5% glucose in water via a peripheral vein for 2–

6 h. The dose of insulin and glucagon administered in the study was arbitrarily chosen, based on previous experimental and clinical data[9,10]. This treatment was repeated three times daily. Patients in the control group received 5% glucose in an identical fashion. Human albumin (2 g) was added to the bottles containing insulin and glucagon to prevent adsorption of the hormones to the infusion set, and to the control bottles to maintain identical appearance of the solutions. The treatment period lasted 3 weeks in the survival cases. Data sheets were collected by the study centre.

Fisher's exact test was used to evaluate the differences in mortality between the two groups and Student's t-test was used for the mean differences.

RESULTS

Table 8.2 shows the characteristics of the patients who were studied. There was no significant difference between the control and the treatment groups concerning sex and age (Table 8.2). The mean alcoholic intake before the diagnosis of alcoholic hepatitis was 176 ± 58 g d^{-1} during a mean period of 16.1 ± 8.2 years. In total, the patients consumed an average of 1028 ± 169 kg alcohol during their lives before the diagnosis of alcoholic hepatitis was made. The duration of excessive alcohol intake was longer and the total amount of ingested alcohol was greater in males (1352 ± 178 kg) than in females (704 ± 151 kg).

The main clinical and biochemical findings of the two groups show similar data (Table 8.3) before the treatment period. In accordance with the clinical and biochemical data, the morphological examination of the liver biopsy material showed severe acute alcoholic hepatitis: hepatocytes with ballooning degeneration with or without Mallory's hyalin, cellular necrosis and infiltration by polymorphonuclear leukocytes. The cellular damage and inflammation affected all zones of the hepatic acinus. In the 51 cases of histologically established alcoholic hepatitis, fatty degeneration of the liver was found in 12 cases, portal fibrosis with increased fibrous tissue in the portal tract in 15 patients, and cirrhosis of the liver with presence of fibrosis surrounding regenerative nodules or pseudo-nodules was observed in the remaining 24 patients. No statistically significant differences in age and clinical features were observed between the sexes at diagnosis. However, the disturbances of liver function tests, as well as the histological severity of alcoholic hepatitis, were greater in females than in males.

A statistically significant difference was found in the rate of survival time (Table 8.4). In the total group of 66 individuals, 19 patients died during this study, 14 in the control group and five in the therapy group ($p \pm 0.05$). Hepatic encephalopathy, characterized by an abnormal mental status, occurred in several cases. The clinical manifestations ranged from a slightly altered mental

114

Table 8.2   Characteristics of patients in the study

	Control (n = 33)	Insulin and glucagon (n = 33)	Total number of cases (n = 66)
Female	15	13	28
Male	18	20	38
Mean age (years ± SD)	46 ± 9	47 ± 12	46.5 ± 10
Number of days before entry into the study (mean ± SD)	4 ± 4	5 ± 3	4.5 ± 3

Table 8.3   Clinical and biochemical findings at time of entry into the study (values are means ± SD)

	Control (n = 33)	Insulin and glucagon (n = 33)
Varices	10	9
Hepatomegaly	21	20
Splenomegaly	9	8
Spider angiomas	7	7
Encephalopathy	10	9
Ascites	5	6
Total bilirubin (μmol L^{-1})	266 ± 40	256 ± 36
Aspartate aminotransferase (U L^{-1})	150 ± 46	138 ± 53
Alanine aminotransferase (U L^{-1})	278 ± 80	302 ± 54
γ-Glutamyltranspeptidase (U L^{-1})	142 ± 32	138 ± 40
Prothrombin time (%)	47 ± 10	49 ± 11

Table 8.4   The effect of insulin and glucagon therapy on the survival rate

	Control group	Treated group
Total patients studied	33	33
No. who survived	19	28*
No. who died	14	5

* In comparison with control groups $p < 0.05$

status to coma. The neuromuscular complications ranged from incoordination and tremor to ophthalmoplegia and incontinence. The symptoms of hepatic coma were directly related to the rapidity with which hepatic coma developed and to its severity. Hepatic encephalopathy with coma led to the death of 11 patients (three of the treatment group and eight of the control group). Oesophageal varix rupture caused death in five cases (two of the treatment group and three of the control group). Lethal bleeding developed from gastric ulcer in one case, and another two patients from the control group died from

Table 8.5 Complications in 19 patients with alcoholic hepatitis who died

	Control group	Insulin and glucagon group
Coma hepaticum (hepatic encepha-	8	3
lopathy)	3	2
Oesophageal varix rupture	1	0
Bleeding from gastric ulcer	2	0
Heart failure		

heart failure (Table 8.5). Of the 19 patients who died, all but one underwent autopsy. The diagnosis of alcoholic hepatitis, which had not been established previously by biopsy in 12 of these 18 patients, was confirmed in all cases.

The changes in the selected laboratory data performed at 10-day intervals during the study are shown in Figures 8.1–8.5. In the control group there was no significant difference between the baseline and final results except for serum bilirubin levels. After the insulin and glucagon treatment, a significant improvement could be demonstrated in the selected biochemical examinations compared with the baseline data and with data found in the control group at the end of the treatment period. The concentration of bilirubin (Figure 8.1) and the activities of AST (Figure 8.2), ALT (Figure 8.3), and GGT (Figure 8.4) in serum decreased, while prothrombin time increased significantly (Figure 8.5) after 3 weeks of therapy. It is important to note that all the parameters except ALT showed a significant improvement only after the three weeks of therapy with insulin and glucagon.

Two patients from the treatment group developed hypoglycaemia. Both of them responded to infusion of 40% dextrose and could be maintained in the trial. The hypoglycaemic episode recurred again in one case, and this time also it was treated with 40% dextrose infusion. Subsequently all the patients were carefully observed during the first few days of infusion and blood sugar measurements were made frequently in venous blood by clinical laboratory means or on finger blood specimens by Dextrostix. After insulin and glucagon infusion fever developed in two cases, nausea and vomiting in another two cases, and in one case the signs of ileus appeared on the fifth day of infusion. The passage became normal after discontinuation of treatment. In the control group nausea and vomiting occurred only in one case after the glucose infusion.

DISCUSSION

The results of the present study show a statistically significant benefit with respect to survival in patients with acute alcoholic hepatitis treated with infusions of insulin and glucagon. The results also demonstrate improvement

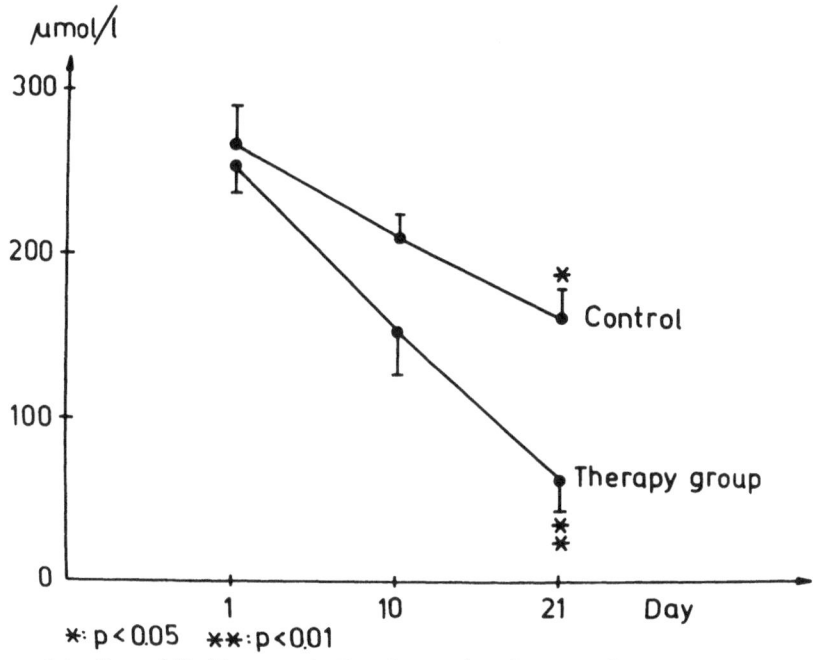

Figure 8.1   Serum bilirubin concentration after insulin–glucagon infusion therapy

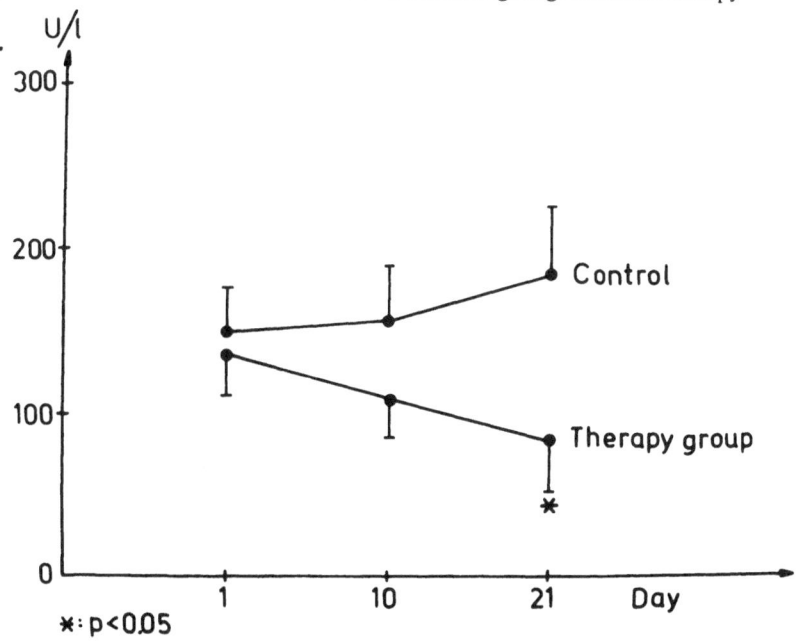

Figure 8.2   Serum aspartate aminotransferase activity after insulin–glucagon infusion therapy

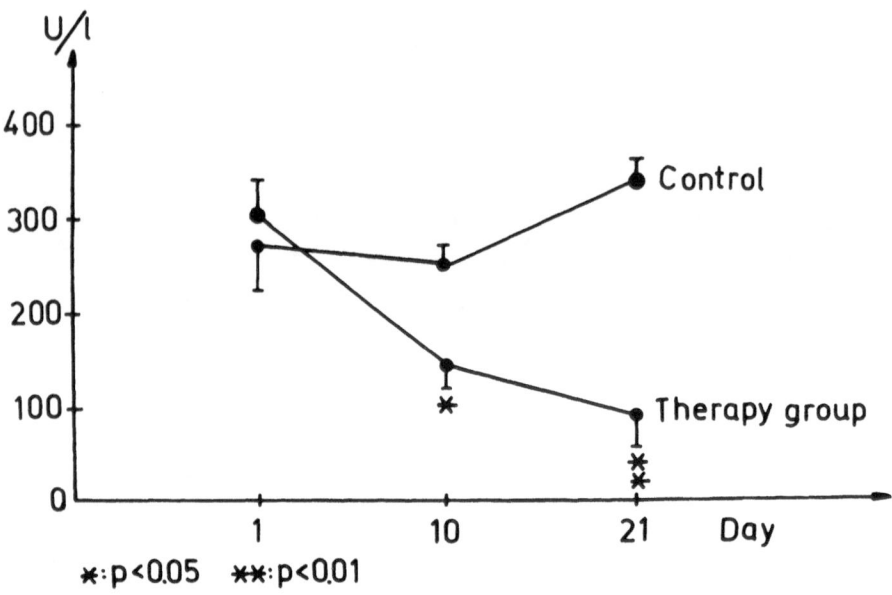

Figure 8.3 Serum alanine aminotransferase activity after insulin–glucagon therapy

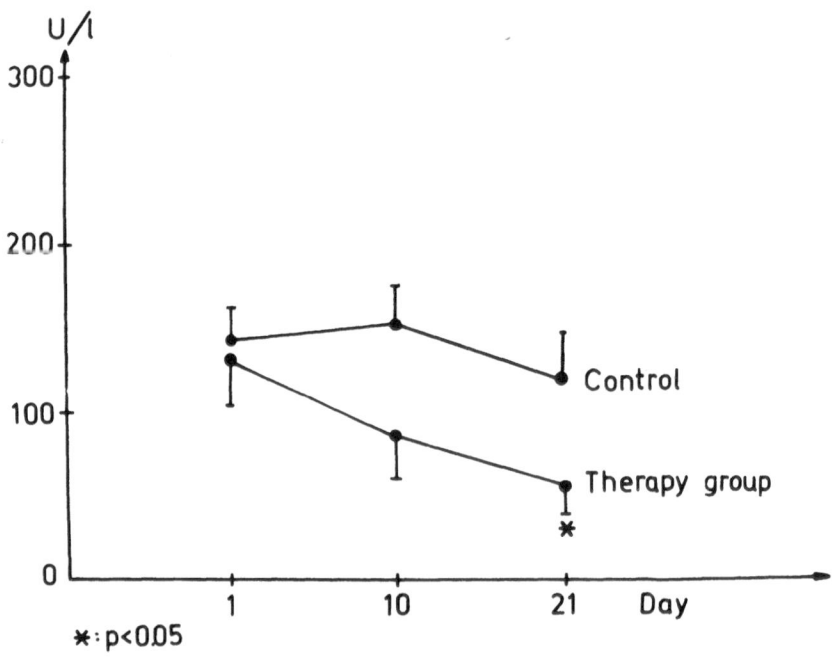

Figure 8.4 Serum γ-glutamyltranspeptidase activity after insulin–glucagon infusion therapy

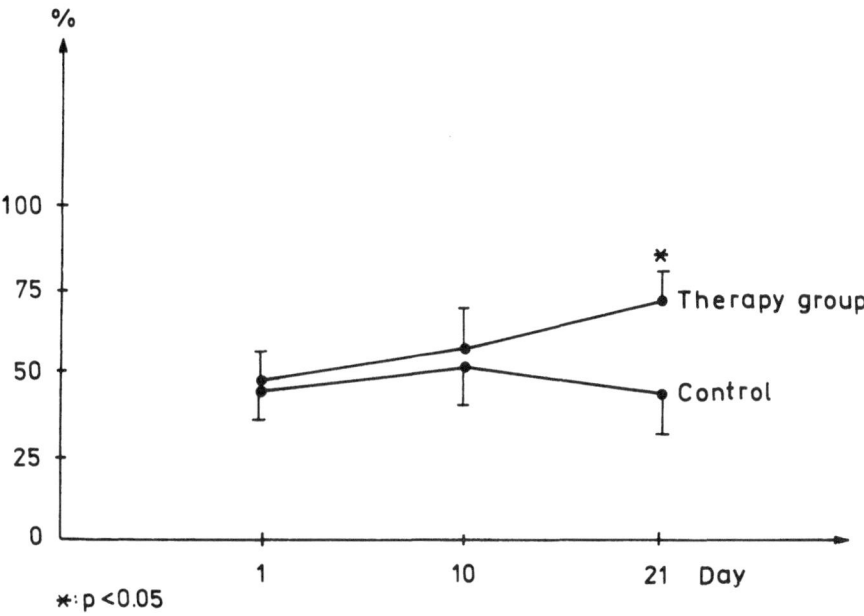

Figure 8.5 Changes in prothrombin time after insulin–glucagon infusion therapy

in selected liver chemistry tests in surviving patients. These findings extend the observations previously reported by Baker et al.[13] where only a trend toward improvement in mortality could be demonstrated in their randomized controlled trial, which included fifty patients. However, one additional study of this treatment in alcoholic hepatitis patients, published only in abstract form from the University of Southern California[14], failed to demonstrate a benefit in treated patients.

The reasons for the better results in our study are not entirely clear. The number of patients investigated was somewhat larger than in the series from the University of Chicago[13]; a larger number of patients in the latter investigation might have yielded statistically significant results. In addition, there may have been differences in the pattern of alcohol consumption, associated nutritional deficits, or the response of the liver to insulin and glucagon between American and Hungarian patients. It is important to note that the protocol for administration of insulin and glucagon differed in our study. We infused insulin and glucagon over 4–6 h, three times daily, for 3 weeks, whereas the American investigators gave the infusion over 12 h daily. Short, repeated courses of treatment may exert a more beneficial effect on the liver. Oka et al.[15], using a protocol similar to ours, found a beneficial effect of insulin and glucagon infusion in severe viral hepatitis. Although mortality was not significantly improved in this study, the patients investigated probably had a relatively low risk of mortality, so that a beneficial effect on mortality might have been missed.

The mechanism by which insulin and glucagon may beneficially influence the mortality of patients with acute alcoholic hepatitis is unknown but, based upon experimental data, stimulation of cell division and hepatic regeneration would appear to be the most likely[13]. Insulin and glucagon probably act as hepatotrophic substances in humans, as previously suggested by several animal studies[16]. Experimental liver disorders of various origins could be inhibited by combined insulin and glucagon treatment[12,17].

There are two additional interesting questions to discuss concerning the present data: the assessment of liver injury, and the higher susceptibility of women to alcoholic liver lesion.

Determining the synthetic capacity of the liver is of considerable clinical value in assessing the severity of acute liver failure[18]. As the liver is the major site of synthesis of blood clotting factors, coagulation abnormalities could serve as indicators of the degree of liver necrosis as well as markers of liver regeneration. When comparing prothrombin time and Factor VII with other markers (prealbumin, fibrinogen, α-fetoprotein), neither one of those provided reliable information, while Factor VII and prothrombin time were equally sensitive. Important to notice is the fact that there is a time lag of approximately 7 days before Factor VII and prothrombin time start to increase. This is probably due to the fact that during the first week the liver synthesis is aimed primarily at the assemblage of structural proteins. In our patients, the prothrombin time did not change significantly during the first period (10 days) but later, in accordance with data in the literature, an increase was found in the prothrombin time of patients treated with insulin and glucagon infusion, reflecting an improved liver function.

Several reports have emphasized the higher risk for women of developing alcoholic liver disease[3,5,6]. Women tend to present with more severe disease than men, even after a shorter period of excessive drinking and a lower daily alcohol consumption. The cause of this sex-related susceptibility to alcohol may be due to differences in body composition, since the volume of distribution of alcohol is smaller in women due to their greater proportion of adipose tissue[6] and to hormonal effects[19]. At diagnosis, the women included in the present series had a lower prothrombin index and more severe enzyme alterations and histological damage than men, indicating a more severe liver disease, although the duration of alcoholism and the cumulative alcohol intake were lower than in men. The total alcohol consumption in women was about half of that found in men. Our results confirm that alcoholic hepatitis is more severe in women.

In conclusion, further studies will be required to determine the mechanism of the beneficial effect of insulin and glucagon infusion therapy in alcoholic hepatitis. Whatever the explanation, the present results suggest that insulin and glucagon infusions should now be considered for the treatment of acute alcoholic hepatitis.

Acknowledgement

This work was supported in part by Novo Industri A/S, Regional Office Eastern Europe, Wien, Austria.

References

1. Sherlock S. Alcohol related liver disease. *Br Med Bull* 1982; 38: 67–70.
2. Fehér J. Pathogenesis and prognosis of chronic active hepatitis. PhD Thesis, Semmelweis University of Budapest, 1980.
3. Sherlock S. Nutrition and alcoholics. *Lancet* 1984; 1: 436–438.
4. Phillips BG, Davidson GS. Acute hepatic insufficiency of chronic alcoholic. *Arch Int Med* 1954; 94: 585–603.
5. Galambos JT. Natural history of alcoholic hepatitis. Part 3. Histological changes. *Gastroenterology* 1972; 63: 1026–1035.
6. Pares A, Caballeria J, Bruguera M, Rodés J. Histological course of alcoholic hepatitis. Influence of abstinence, sex, and extent of hepatic damage. *J Hepatol* 1986; 2: 33–42.
7. Porter HP, Simon RF, Pope CE, Vollwiler W, Fenster LF. Corticosteroid therapy in severe alcoholic hepatitis: A double blind drug trial. *N Engl J Med* 1971; 284: 1350–1355.
8. Maddrey WC, Boinott JK, Bedine MS, Weber FL, Mezey E, White RI. Corticosteroid therapy of alcoholic hepatitis. *Gastroenterology* 1978; 75: 193–199.
9. Dölle W. Drug therapy in liver disease. *Hepatology Rapid Literature Review, Freiburg* 1985; 6: 11–12.
10. Tescke R, Matrini GA, Strohmeyer G. Was ist gesichert in der Therapie toxisch bedinger Lebererkrankungen? *Internist* 1983; 24: 690–698.
11. Fehér J, Láng I, Nékám K, Csomós G, Müzes G, Deák G. Effect of silibinin on the activity and expression of superoxide dismutase (SOD) in lymphocytes from patients with chronic alcoholic liver disease. *Free Radical Res Commun* 1987; in press.
12. Farivar M, Wands JR, Isselbacher KJ, Bucher NLR. Effect of insulin and glucagon on fulminant murine hepatitis. *N Engl J Med* 1976; 295: 1517–1519.
13. Baker AL, Jaspan JB, Haines NW, Hatfield GE, Krager PS, Schneider JF. A randomized clinical trial of insulin and glucagon infusion for treatment of alcoholic hepatitis: A progress report in 50 patients. *Gastroenterology* 1981; 80: 1410–1414.
14. Radvan G, Kanel G, Redeker A. Insulin and glucagon infusion in acute alcoholic hepatitis. *Gastroenterology* 1982; 82: 1154.
15. Oka H, Okita K, Fujiwara K. Glucagon and insulin therapy in fulminant hepatic failure in Japan. In: Picazo J, ed. *Glucagon in Gastroenterology and Hepatology*. Lancaster: MTP Press, 1982: 171–178.
16. Sherlock S. Portal venous 'goodies' and fulminant viral hepatitis. *N Engl J Med* 1976; 295: 1535–1536.
17. Starzl TE, Porter KA, Watanabe K, Putnam CW. Effect of insulin, glucagon, and insulin/glucagon infusions on liver morphology and cell division after complete portacaval shunt in dogs. *Lancet* 1976; 1: 821–825.
18. Farinati F, Pengo V, Bassi N, Naccarato R, D'Amico D. Monitoring liver regeneration after right hepatectomy. *Ital J Surg Sci* 1985; 15: 75–77.
19 Fehér J, Vereckei A. *Free Radical Reactions in Medicine*. Budapest: Biogal-Medicina, 1985.

DISCUSSION

Carr-Locke   Professor Fehér, I have two questions for you. The first one is the basis for the diagnosis of alcoholic hepatitis which is, of course, fundamental to the study. Were you able to biopsy all the patients in your study or not?

Fehér   Yes, of course, we did biopsies in all the patients except 15 in whom biopsies were contraindicated due to prolonged prothrombin time.

Carr-Locke   In that case, can you tell me what proportion of patients also had cirrhosis and was there a difference between the two groups or were none of the patients cirrhotic?

Fehér   Considering cirrhosis, there was no significant difference between the two groups. We did histological examinations in all the cases biopsied and 11 appeared to be cirrhotic among the controls and 13 in the glucagon/insulin treated material. But, furthermore, after autopsy in 19 patients, we were able to see the same histological evidence, and it was this histological data with Mallory bodies, hyaline alterations, and granulocytic infiltrations, coupled with a history of high alcohol consumption that led us to confirm the diagnosis of alcoholic hepatitis.

Fujiwara   I wonder if there was a difference in the patients' appetite between both groups.

Fehér   No, there was no difference between the two groups in the case of appetite.

Nikolov   I would like to ask you whether it is necessary to use insulin plus glucagon, because I see that there is a generalized tendency to use them combined, but you have no studies with a separate insulin group and a separate group with glucagon ...

Fehér   Well, in the first place, according to the available literature, mainly Dr Baker's data, and also from animal experiments and from *in vitro* studies with hepatocytes, it is assumed that using glucagon together with insulin is better for cell regeneration. In the second place, it is my hypothesis that glucagon acts as a scavenger, a free-radical scavenger, and that insulin is necessary in order for glucose to be able to penetrate the cells when there are alterations in the liver membrane coming from the pathologically high number of free radicals, for instance superoxide anions, hydroxyl anions, hydroxyl radicals, etc. In this case, glucagon is able to scavenge these pathologically increased superoxide anions in the plasma membrane. Before, I asked Professor Lefèbvre about calcium metabolism. I believe there is some relativity with calcium metabolism and this effect of glucagon. As a matter of fact, we have performed some new experiments with glucagon/insulin in an *in vitro* study by which we wanted to know the separate effect of glucagon and insulin on cell migration with granulocyte cultures and on lymphokine production. In granulocytes the migration area did not change during glucagon concentration. Migration inhibition was not altered after using glucagon, and the same was found after using insulin. However, if we use lymphocytes for the production of lymphokine, we do observe an inhibition of the migration of granulocytes. After using glucagon alone, insulin alone, and glucagon together with insulin in the incubation material all of them were able to produce an inhibition in the case of lymphokine production. From these experiments we can expect that glucagon, insulin, and glucagon and insulin together may be able to act in the case of lymphocyte and granulocyte interaction, and therefore in the future we would like to carry out these experiments in lymphocytes and granulocytes from patients with acute alcoholic liver diseases.

Vilardell One thing that has surprised me a little is that the γ-GT values that you have presented are a bit low in comparison to what we see in our own hospital. γ-GT values of a little over 200 are not as high as what we generally see ...

Fehér In some cases we saw γ-GT values of 600 or more in cases of alcoholic liver cirrhosis and alcoholic liver steatosis, but in the cases of acute alcoholic hepatitis, the γ-glutamyl transpeptidase values we have seen, are not as high in the cases of alcoholic liver cirrhosis and in alcoholic liver steatosis. I do not know the cause, but I must say that this is really a very thorough observation from our material.

Vilardell Another thing that I would like to point out which seems striking to me is the mortality rate that you reported for both groups. If you exclude the patients who died from bleeding, from portal hypertension, etc., do you still get a statistical difference?

Fehér Yes, we do.

Nikolov Why do you not use lactic dehydrogenase as a parameter for measurement?

Fehér The reason is only a question of economy. But, at any rate, according to the literature in 90% of cases, three parameters are enough to make a diagnosis, that is why we have used these three parameters and no more.

Carr-Locke Your study lasted 3 weeks, is that right?

Fehér Three weeks, that is right.

Carr-Locke Can you tell us the survival rate of your patients after 3 weeks?

Fehér I do not know the exact number of patients who died, because some of the patients who survived initially died later on, but there was a very unusual case of one patient who had alcoholic hepatitis five times. This patient was involved in the study on one of these five occasions, and was given glucose infusion without glucagon and insulin which brought her very near to death. This is just one example of the benefit of treatment of acute alcoholic hepatitis.

9
Clinical evaluation of glucagon–insulin therapy for acute hepatitis severe form

H. OKA, K. FUJIWARA, K. OKITA, H. ISHII and A. SAKUMA

INTRODUCTION

Bucher et al.[1] have reported the synergistic hepatotrophic action of glucagon and insulin in eviscerated partially hepatectomized rats. Likewise, Farivar et al.[2] also demonstrated that mortality is reduced in mice infected with murine hepatitis virus when both glucagon and insulin are administered.

These experimental studies suggest that the infusion of glucagon and insulin might be effective in the treatment of acute liver injury in humans. In this connection, Baker et al.[3,4] reported on a clinical trial in which combined infusions of glucagon and insulin were used in the treatment of alcoholic hepatitis.

In Japan, combined infusions of glucagon and insulin have been used clinically for fulminant hepatic failure since 1977[5]. The survival rate of patients with fulminant hepatic failure treated with this therapy has been found to be higher than that of untreated patients, suggesting a possible benefit of this therapy[6]. The importance of proving the value of therapies by conducting controlled studies is evident. For this reason, we conducted a multicentre double-blind controlled trial of this therapy in connection with hepatitis. However, this study was conducted in patients with a severe type of acute hepatitis since, for us, the performance of such a trial in patients with fulminant hepatic failure would hardly be acceptable from an ethical point of view.

METHODS

The patients chosen were those with acute hepatitis with a prothrombin time between 30 and 60% of the normal value, hepaplastin test between 30 and 50%, or thrombotest 30 to 50%. Patients with hepatic coma (grade III or more) or other severe complications such as malignancies, gastrointestinal bleeding, severe infection or disseminated intravascular coagulation, and those over 70 years of age, were excluded. Insulin-dependent diabetic patients were also excluded. Likewise, patients treated with glucocorticoids, fresh plasma, amino-acid infusions, or other special therapeutic measures were also excluded.

After obtaining informed consent to enter the study, patients were randomly assigned to the glucagon-insulin group or to the placebo group. The doses of glucagon and insulin used were 1 mg and 10 units, respectively. The hormones were dissolved in 500 ml of 5% glucose solution and infused twice daily for 1 week. The placebo group patients received 5% glucose solution according to a similar schedule. From July 1981 to March 1985, 98 patients entered the study, 51 into the glucagon-insulin group and 47 into the placebo group.

Liver function tests including prothrombin time, hepaplastin test or thrombotest and α-fetoprotein, and measurement of serum electrolytes, were performed on admission to the study, on the fourth day of treatment, and every week thereafter for 4 weeks. Fasting blood levels were determined every morning during the treatment period, and weekly thereafter. The global improvement rating, overall safety rating, and global utility rating, were evaluated by the physicians in charge based on the changes in clinical signs and laboratory data and adverse effects of the treatment.

RESULTS AND DISCUSSION

The clinical backgrounds of the patients studied are shown in Table 9.1. About two-thirds of the patients were male, and three quarters of the cases in both groups had hepatitis of viral origin. The distribution of the patients regarding sex, age, and hepatitis aetiology was not significantly different. However, the patients in the glucagon–insulin group were somewhat older than those in the placebo group, that is, the number of patients over 50 years in the glucagon–insulin group was greater than in the placebo group. Of the 98 patients who comprised the study, eight patients were excluded from the utility analysis, five because they were found to have liver cirrhosis following liver biopsy, and three for which no liver function tests were available for the treatment and post-treatment periods. These eight cases, and six patients who were treated for only 1 day, were excluded from the global improvement analysis. The global improvement rating of each patient was evaluated according to a score ('100 points' as full mark) by the physician in charge, and the study steering committee decided that patients with scores of 70 points or more

Table 9.1   Clinical backgrounds of patients studied

	Glucagon–insulin treated group	Placebo group
No. of cases	51	47
Male	35 (68.6)[a]	30 (63.8)
Female	16 (31.4)	17 (36.2)
Age in years: 10–19	1	2
20–29	13	12
30–39	9	13
40–49	7	11
50–59	12	6
60–69	6	2
70–79	3	1
Viral hepatitis: A type	10 (19.6)	12 (25.5)
B type	19 (37.3)	14 (29.8)
non-A non-B type	7 (13.7)	11 (23.4)
Drug-induced hepatitis	5 (9.8)	3 (6.4)
Alcoholic hepatitis	3 (5.9)	6 (12.8)
Aetiology unknown	7 (13.7)	1 (2.1)

[a] % values in parentheses
Differences were not significant (Wilcoxon test)

were to be evaluated as improved. Of 42 treated cases, 34 (81.0%) were rated as improved, while out of 42 cases in the placebo group, 28 (66.7%) showed improvement. This difference was not statistically significant.

Adverse effects were observed in 25 cases of the glucagon-insulin group and four cases of the placebo group. The main symptoms leading to discontinuation of the infusion were nausea and vomiting. Hypoglycaemia was observed in 11 cases of the glucagon–insulin group, and one case of the placebo group. Two of the patients in the former group developing hypoglycaemia had blood sugar levels under 40 mg ml^{-1}. Hypoglycaemia was treated by an infusion of glucose solution and both patients recovered. The incidence of infusion-related symptoms such as hypoglycaemia, nausea and vomiting was significantly more frequent in the glucagon–insulin group (Table 9.2).

Based on the global improvement rating and the adverse effects of treatment, the utility rating for each patient was assessed by the physicians in charge and scores of 65 points or more were considered as indicators of usefulness of the therapy. Of 46 cases treated with the glucagon–insulin infusions, 24 were rated as treatment having been useful, while infusions were also rated as treatment having been useful in half of the cases of the placebo group.

The levels of serum transaminases decreased rapidly during treatment, and returned to almost normal levels 1 or 2 weeks after treatment in both groups (Figure 9.1), indicating that patients were at the recovery stage of acute

Table 9.2   Adverse effects after treatment

	Glucagon–insulin treated group	Placebo group
No. of cases	51	47
Total no. of cases with symptoms	25 (49.0)[a]*	4 (8.5)
Hypoglycaemia	11 (21.6)*	1 (2.1)
Nausea	11 (21.6)*	1 (2.1)
Vomiting	11 (21.6)*	0
Sweating	3 (5.9)	2 (4.3)
Anorexia	3 (5.9)	0
Palpitation	2 (3.9)	0
Discomfort	2 (3.9)	0
Others	5 (9.8)	3 (6.4)
No. of symptoms	48	7

[a] % values in parentheses
* In comparison with placebo group $p < 0.001$; other differences were not significant

hepatitis when the infusion therapy was started. There were no differences in these parameters between the two groups.

Serum total and direct bilirubin levels started to decrease several days after the beginning of treatment in both groups. Though the mean bilirubin levels in patients from the glucagon–insulin group were slightly higher than those in patients of the placebo group, the rates of improvement were similar in both groups (Figure 9.2).

The changes of serum total protein and albumin levels during and after treatment are shown in Figure 9.3. In the glucagon–insulin group, the mean values of serum total protein and albumin were lower than those in the placebo group during and after treatment. Serum albumin levels decreased during treatment and thereafter rapidly increased up to a normal value. The rates of improvement of these parameters after treatment were not different between the two groups. Serum total cholesterol levels increased rapidly during and after treatment in both groups. An increase of α-fetoprotein levels, which was maintained up to the second week after treatment, was observed in patients of the glucagon–insulin group, but the differences between the values before and after treatment were not significant. Likewise, the differences between both groups were not significant, since α-fetoprotein values were very variable (Figure 9.4).

The prothrombin time changes during and after treatment are shown in Figure 9.5. Although the prolongation of prothrombin time tended to be greater in the glucagon–insulin group than in the placebo group when the therapy was started, the recovery after treatment was more rapid in the glucagon–insulin group and, consequently, the rate of improvement was significantly greater for the treated cases 1 and 2 weeks after treatment. Since

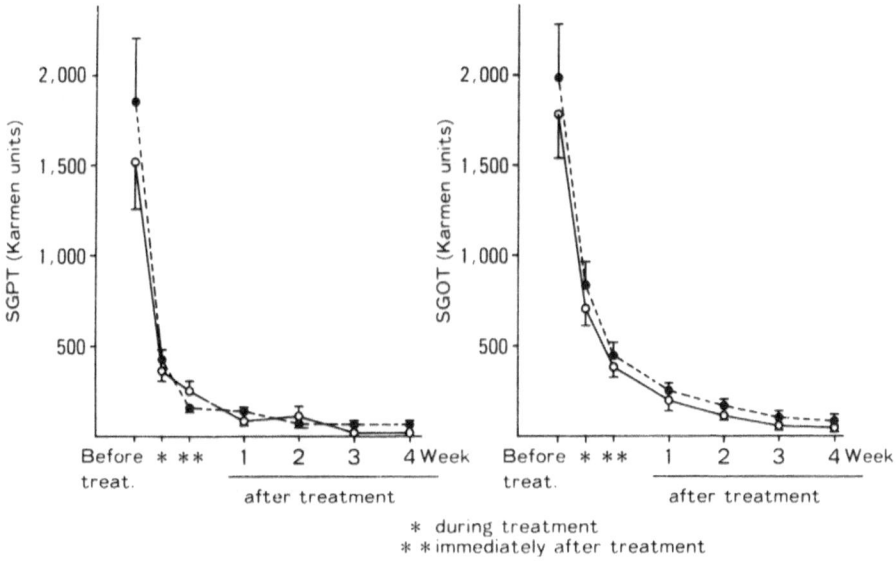

Figure 9.1 Changes in SGOT and SGPT values during and after treatment. SGOT and SGPT were measured on the day of admission, fourth day of treatment, immediately after treatment and every week thereafter. Open circles indicate glucagon–insulin infusion group, closed circles placebo group

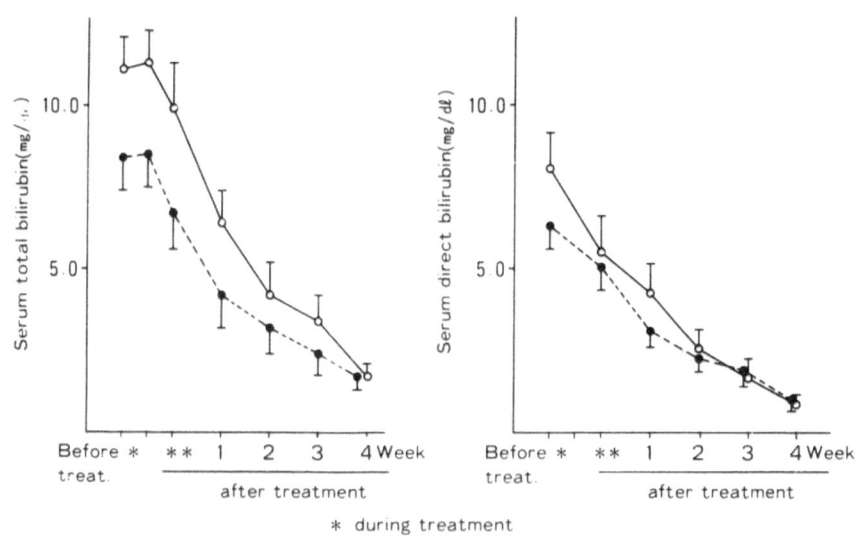

Figure 9.2 Changes in serum total and direct bilirubin values during and after treatment. Open circles indicate glucagon–insulin infusion group, closed circles placebo group

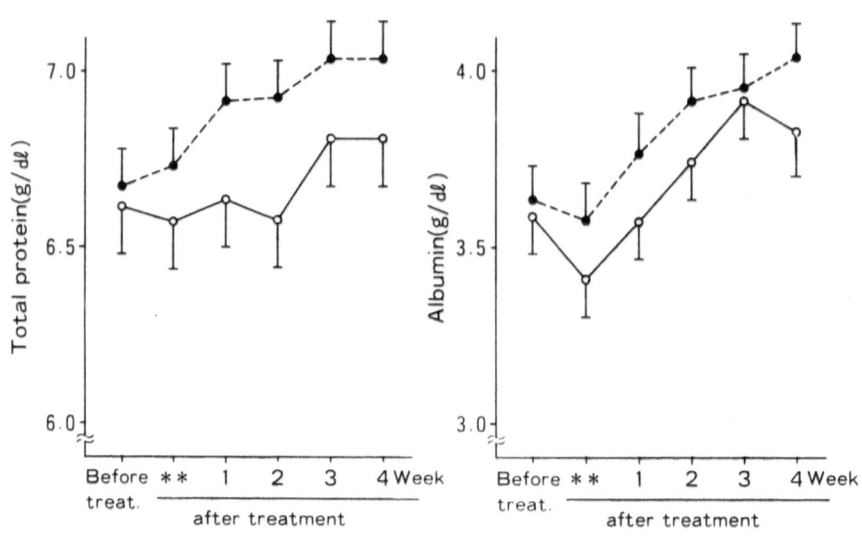

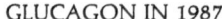

Figure 9.3 Changes in serum total protein and albumin values during and after treatment. Open circles indicate glucagon–insulin infusion group, closed circles placebo group

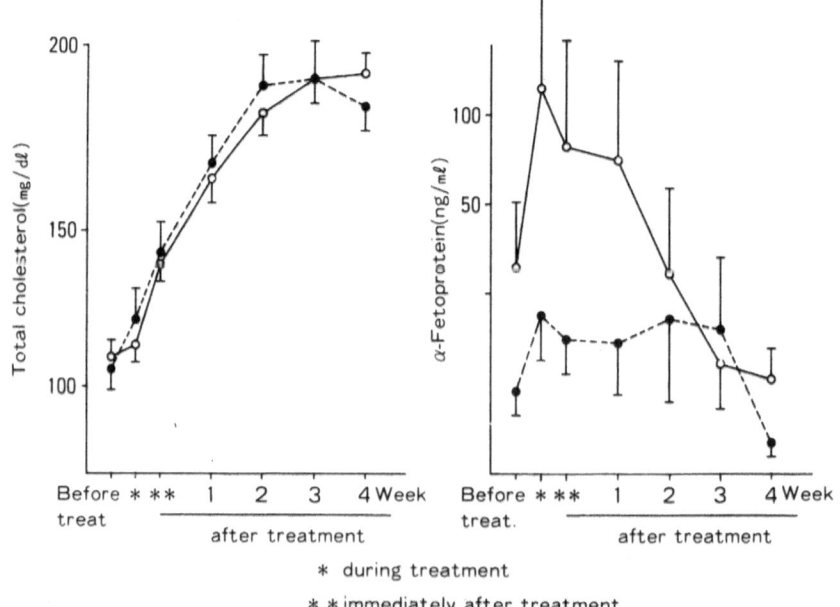

Figure 9.4 Changes in serum total cholesterol and α-fetoprotein values during and after treatment. Open circles indicate glucagon–insulin infusion group, closed circles placebo group

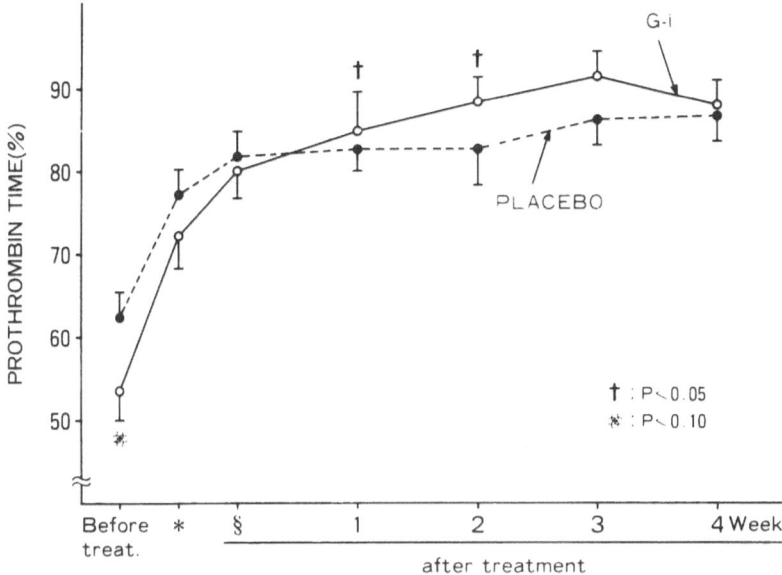

Figure 9.5 Changes in prothrombin time (%) during and after treatment. Prothrombin time (%) in the glucagon–insulin infusion (G-I) group was somewhat lower than that in the placebo group, but the difference is not significant

prothrombin time is assumed to be the most sensitive parameter for protein synthesis in the liver, this change may result from the stimulation by glucagon and insulin of liver cell proliferation or recovery from injury.

In summary, the infusion of glucagon and insulin did not affect the global improvement rating in patients with a severe type of acute hepatitis. Adverse effects such as hypoglycaemia, nausea and vomiting were observed in 21.6% of the cases, although those were not severe. Thus, the clinical benefit of this therapy for the treatment of patients with a severe form of acute hepatitis was not confirmed in this study. However, the infusion of glucagon and insulin tended to elevate α-fetoprotein levels and significantly stimulated the recovery of prolonged prothrombin time in these patients, suggesting a stimulating effect of this therapy on liver regeneration or on the recovery from liver injury.

References

1. Bucher NLR, Swaffield MN. Regulation of hepatic regeneration in rats by synergistic action of insulin and glucagon. *Proc Natl Acad Sci USA* 1987; 72: 1157–1160.
2. Farivar M, Wands JR, Isselbacher KJ, Bucher NLR. Effect of insulin and glucagon on fulminant murine hepatitis. *N Engl J Med* 1976; 295: 1517–1519.
3. Baker AL, Jaspan JB, Haines NW, Hatfield GE, Krager PS, Schneider JF. A randomized clinical trial of insulin and glucagon infusion for treatment of alcoholic hepatitis. Progress report in 50 patients. *Gastroenterology* 1981; 80: 1410–1414.

4. Baker AL. Insulin and glucagon for liver disease. Assessment of response in patients with alcoholic hepatitis. In: Picazo J, ed. *Glucagon in Gastroenterology and Hepatology.* Lancaster: MTP Press, 1982: 155–169.
5. Okiita K, Matsuda S, Hata K, Morimoto T, Sasaki M, Fukumoto Y, Kodama T, Takemoto T. Clinical use of glucagon and insulin in therapy of fulminant hepatic failure. *Gastroenterol Jpn* 1979; 14: 453–457.
6. Oka H, Okita K, Fujiwara K, Glucagon and insulin therapy in fulminant hepatic failure in Japan. In: Picazo J, ed. *Glucagon in Gastroenterology and Hepatology.* Lancaster: MTP Press, 1982: 171–180.

DISCUSSION

Fehér   Professor Oka, I should like to ask you about your data concerning the histological alterations of the liver because I find that these were very mild in the cases you have reported. I think that glucagon/insulin/glucose infusion therapy is more effective in the severe form of liver diseases, specially in the severe toxic form, and not as effective in the case of acute hepatitis, so could you please explain this?

Oka   Yes. In the first place, this was a histological examination where only a few cases were able to undergo biopsy since most of the patients in this study had acute hepatitis. On the other hand we think that perhaps the injury of acute hepatitis is able to recover spontaneously, so actually what we tried to see in this study was if there was an effect of glucagon and insulin on protein synthesis as a liver function in the case of injured liver.

Baker   I would like to ask you a mechanical question about the analysis of your data, Professor Oka. You have shown us the difference in prothrombin time between the glucagon/insulin treated patients and the control patients. What kind of statistical analysis was that, was it analysis of variance?

Oka   For prothrombin time we used the paired *t*-test measuring the difference between the values obtained at the start of treatment and those from 1 week after treatment and, as I have shown, the difference proved to be significantly higher in the glucagon/insulin group.

Baker   The more important question I have for you really is about your attitude towards a randomized controlled trial in the most severe forms of hepatitis, fulminant hepatic failure. Has the experience that you and other Japanese investigators have had with this severe form of hepatitis, which is not of the most severe type, made you interest yourselves in doing a trial in fulminant hepatic failure?

Oka   As you know, acute hepatic failure has a very poor prognosis and, at least in Japan, most doctors agree about not performing double control studies in such cases. That is why we did the study only in patients with the severe form of acute hepatitis. But as soon as we see the patient progress to hepatic failure which may lead to hepatic coma, this patient is automatically excluded from the study. So answering your question, due to this ethical problem it is quite impossible to perform such a type of study with glucagon/insulin in the most severe forms of fulminant hepatic failure.

Skucas   The question that occurs to me naturally here is if there is any difference in the response between the alcoholic hepatitis patients and the viral hepatitis patients. I do realize Professor Oka that you only have some patients with alcoholic hepatitis in your group, but do these patients respond to glucagon/insulin treatment predominantly one way or the other?

Oka   In our material the response of the patients with alcoholic hepatitis was almost the same as those with viral hepatitis.

Vilardell   So you did not find any difference really between the sub-groups you studied?

Oka   No, we did not, but as I said, we only had a few patients with alcoholic hepatitis. That is why there was no statistical difference between the placebo group and the glucagon/insulin group.

Vilardell   One thing that I find really interesting is to realize that more and more we are being able to see or at least diagnose so many cases of severe hepatitis A, as Professor Oka has shown here, while before we thought it was something else. I think it is really an important difference to be able to make a prognosis knowing whether a disease is benign or not.

Baker   An additional question that I have for you Professor Oka has to do with the data you showed with the α-fetoprotein. Certainly one of the problems in the use of glucagon and insulin for the treatment of liver disease or any other new treatment for this indication is to be able to identify the patients who are the most likely to respond. Do you think of α-fetoprotein as a good marker of responsiveness or have you studied any other markers of responsiveness that you think we could use in future studies such as this?

Oka   Yes, I think that α-fetoprotein is a marker of regeneration from liver injury and that is why we measured it.

10
Clinical evaluation of glucagon and insulin in therapy of fulminant hepatitis

K. OKITA, S. MATSUDA and T. TAKEMOTO

INTRODUCTION

Fulminant hepatitis (FH) is defined as a clinical syndrome that develops as a result of massive necrosis of liver cells followed by severe impairment of hepatic function due to viral infection or drugs, in a patient in whom there has been no previous evidence of liver disease. The mortality rate of this condition is extremely high[1-3]. A nationwide survey conducted in Japan comprising the period 1974–1976, when steroid hormone and/or blood exchange was believed to be useful, revealed a 16.5% survival in FH cases[4].

In principle, treatment of FH should be based on enhancing the liver's regenerating capacity. Recent *in vivo* and *in vitro* studies on liver regeneration have shown important roles for epidermal growth factor, glucagon and insulin as the signals for the trigger mechanism leading to liver regeneration[5-12]. On this basis, it might be recommended that patients presenting with massive liver necrosis should be treated with glucagon and insulin. We have, therefore, developed a new therapeutic regimen of application of these pancreatic hormones and have evaluated their usefulness in the treatment of FH.

DIAGNOSIS OF FH

The diagnosis of FH is based on the criteria proposed by the 12th Inuyama Symposium which was held in 1981 and accepted by the Study Group of Fulminant Hepatitis: hepatitis indicating hepatic encephalopathy over grade 2, an impaired prothrombin time of less than 40% of the normal value which should have developed within 8 weeks of the onset of symptoms and, from the point of view of prognosis, being classified into two forms, in which encephalopathy develops either within 10 days (acute form) or after 10 days (subacute form).

Regarding prognosis, the nationwide survey revealed a higher survival among the acute form cases[4]. Therefore the therapeutic benefit of glucagon and insulin (G–I) therapy was evaluated for each of the forms in comparison with other therapies.

G–I THERAPY

One mg glucagon (Novo, Denmark) and 10 U regular insulin (Novo, Denmark) were dissolved in 500 mg of 5% glucose solution just before use, and infused via a peripheral vein over periods of 2 to 6 h each time. In the early critical period of FH, two courses of treatment per day were given.

Following G–I therapy, a solution containing a high dose of branched chain amino-acids was infused, because of the remarkable decrease in the branched chain amino-acid (valine + leucine + isoleucine)/aromatic amino acid (phenyl-alanine + tyrosine) molar ratio (Table 10.1), which might be a cause of hepatic encephalopathy[13].

In addition to these therapies, antibiotics for infection, diuretics, and H_2-receptor antagonists for upper gastrointestinal bleeding were used, if needed. Changes in hepatic coma, liver function, renal function, and serum electrolytes were carefully observed.

The therapeutic effect of the simultaneous administration of glucagon and insulin was evaluated in comparison with prednisolone therapy and also with a combination therapy consisting of either blood exchange or plasmapheresis in both groups.

CLINICAL EVALUATION OF G–I THERAPY

Patients studied

Of the 15 FH patients treated with prednisolone, six cases were of acute form and eight cases of subacute form. In this group, 13 of the FH cases were caused by infection with hepatitis virus (HB:4, NANB:9), and two cases by sensitivity reactions to drugs administered in the treatment of conditions other than liver disease (Table 10.2).

Table 10.1 Plasma amino-acid profile in liver diseases (μmol L^{-1}; means $\pm$ SD, n in parentheses)

	Normal (8)	Cirrhosis Comp. (5)	Cirrhosis Decomp. (8)	Hepatitis Acute (3)	Hepatitis Fulminant (5)
Thr	146 ± 40	122 ± 25	169 ± 87	140 ± 3	631 ± 460
Ser	214 ± 128	149 ± 9	189 ± 64	182 ± 56	619 ± 514
Asp	102 ± 39	45 ± 32	56 ± 32	43 ± 31	196 ± 187
Gln	610 ± 153	653 ± 113	624 ± 147	495 ± 83	2287 ± 2179
Glu	166 ± 64	165 ± 130	91 ± 54	199 ± 78	310 ± 174
Pro	199 ± 82	148 ± 66	179 ± 51	144 ± 83	753 ± 881
Gly	352 ± 241	219 ± 56	278 ± 67	267 ± 52	1224 ± 1108
Ala	415 ± 70	293 ± 119	347 ± 193	336 ± 753	1685 ± 1233
Val	226 ± 41	170 ± 47	157 ± 27	219 ± 30	499 ± 420
Met	36 ± 10	56 ± 41	89 ± 67	39 ± 14	448 ± 342
Ile	70 ± 16	46 ± 16	45 ± 11	77 ± 18	218 ± 255
Leu	133 ± 35	75 ± 21	71 ± 18	126 ± 14	378 ± 377
Tyr	67 ± 13	152 ± 62	116 ± 53	35 ± 32	251 ± 179
Phe	93 ± 31	74 ± 69	81 ± 41	66 ± 11	316 ± 294
Trp	97 ± 44	50 ± 66	14 ± 27	24 ± 42	74 ± 114
Orn	57 ± 39	79 ± 52	99 ± 41	96 ± 33	417 ± 411
Lys	23 ± 107	151 ± 35	176 ± 56	202 ± 37	1111 ± 1134
His	87 ± 23	69 ± 23	67 ± 13	73 ± 22	338 ± 349
Arg	168 ± 81	167 ± 101	153 ± 69	124 ± 45	629 ± 839
Fischer[a]	4.4 ± 2.7	1.9 ± 1.5	1.6 ± 0.9	4.8 ± 2.6	1.9 ± 1.3

[a] Values for molar ratios of (Val + Leu + Ile)/(Phe + Tyr) taken from ref. 13

On the other hand, of the 38 cases treated with G–I, 17 cases were classified as acute form and the remaining 21 cases as subacute form. In this group, 32 cases of FH were supposed to be due to hepatitis virus (HB:18, NANB:14), and six cases were caused by adverse effects of drugs (Table 10.2).

There were no significant differences in demographic features between the two groups, as shown in Table 10.2. However, there were somewhat worse characteristics in severity of liver dysfunction in the group treated with G–I (Table 10.3).

Therapeutic effect

For ethical reasons, a randomized trial for evaluation of G–I therapy in FH was not performed; very high mortality is associated with this disease. Therefore, the selection of the therapeutic modality was left to the judgement of the physician in charge, after consultation with the patient's family.

Of the 53 cases who entered this study, 14 (26.4%) survived as the result of medication: 13 (34%) of the 38 patients in the G–I group, and one (7%) of the 15 patients in the prednisolone group.

In both groups treated with either prednisolone or simultaneous infusion

Table 10.2 Characteristics of the FH patients studied

	Prednisolone-treated group (n = 15)	Glucagon–insulin-treated group (n = 38)
Female	8 (53[a])	16 (42)
Male	7 (47)	22 (58)
Age in years	37 ± 13[b]	43 ± 15
Aetiology		
hepatitis virus HB	4 (27)	18 (47)
hepatitis virus NANB	9 (60)	14 (37)
adverse effects of drugs	2 (13)	6 (16)
Acute form	6 (40)	17 (45)
Subacute form	9 (60)	21 (55)
Survival	1 (7)	13 (34)*

[a]% values in parentheses; [b]values are means ± SD
* In comparison with prednisolone-treated group, $p < 0.05$

Table 10.3 Liver function parameters on entry into study of patients with acute or subacute forms of FH treated with either prednisolone (PD) or glucagon and insulin (G–I) infusion (values are means ± SD, n in parentheses)

	Acute form		Subacute form	
	PD (6)	G–I (18)	PD (9)	G–I (20)
Albumin (g/dl^{-1})	3.1 ± 0.3	3.0 ± 0.5	2.7 ± 0.2	2.8 ± 0.4
GOT (IU)	2741 ± 948	2152 ± 1686	1151 ± 258	427 ± 534
GPT (IU)	2160 ± 921	1729 ± 1072	918 ± 190	507 ± 570
Bilirubin (mg/dl^{-1})	12.0 ± 3.7	11.4 ± 6.4	12.2 ± 2.4	21.8 ± 15.0
Cholesterol (mg/ml^{-1})	134 ± 19	101 ± 38	139 ± 5	85 ± 36
PTT (%)	15 ± 5	15 ± 4	19 ± 6	14 ± 6

GOT = glutamate-oxaloacetate transaminase; GPT = glutamate-pyruvate transaminase; PTT = prothrombin time

of G–I, combination therapy with blood exchange or plasmapheresis was applied. As shown in Table 10.4, blood exchange was administered to five of the 15 cases treated with prednisolone, while of the 38 patients receiving G–I therapy, five were treated by blood exchange and 12 by plasmapheresis.

In the group treated with prednisolone alone, all 10 cases were fatalities, and of the five cases with combined blood exchange only one patient recovered. With regards to the 38 patients infused with G–I, the following survived: six of the 14 cases treated only with G–I, one of the five cases also having blood exchange, and six of the 19 cases treated together with plasmapheresis.

Concerning the survival rate for each form of FH, in the acute form the

Table 10.4 Survival rates for patients with acute or subacute forms of FH under different therapeutic regimens

	Therapeutic regimen	Survival rate	
Acute form	PD	0/2	(0%)
	PD plus BE	1/4	(25%)
	G–I	4/8	(50%)
	G–I plus BE	1/3	(33%)
	G–I plus PP	4/6	(67%)
Subacute form	PD	0/8	(0%)
	PD plus BE	0/1	(0%)
	G–I	2/6	(33%)
	G–I plus BE	0/2	(0%)
	G–I plus PP	2/13	(15%)

PD = prednisolone; G–I = glucagon and insulin infusion; BE = blood exchange; PP = plasmapheresis

Table 10.5 Comparison of survival periods in groups of FH patients treated with either prednisolone (PD) or glucagon and insulin (G–I) (values are means ± SD)

Treatment	Form of FH	No. of cases	Survival period (days)
PD	Acute	5	4.4 ± 1.7
	Subacute	9	3.4 ± 0.9
	Total	14	3.7 ± 0.9
G–I	Acute	10	6.8 ± 3.8
	Subacute	15	10.5 ± 10.2
	Total	25	8.4 ± 8.2

[a]No significant difference; [b] significant difference, $p < 0.05$; [c]significant difference, $p < 0.05$ (χ^2 test)

combination of simultaneous administration of G–I and plasmapheresis gave the highest survival rate (67%). Therapy with G–I alone resulted in the second highest survival rate (50%). On the other hand, in the subacute form patients treated with G–I without any combination therapies showed a 33% survival rate, and among the cases treated with G–I and other therapies, the survival rate never increased.

Furthermore, the therapeutic effect was evaluated according to the duration of the survival period in the patients who died (Table 10.5). The patients treated with G–I showed a statistically significant prolongation of the survival period, particularly in the subacute form ($p < 0.05$), as compared with the cases given prednisolone, which seems to be neither beneficial nor harmful in the treatment of FH. These results also support the evidence concerning the lack of efficacy of steroid therapy for FH provided by Berk[14] and the EASL report[15].

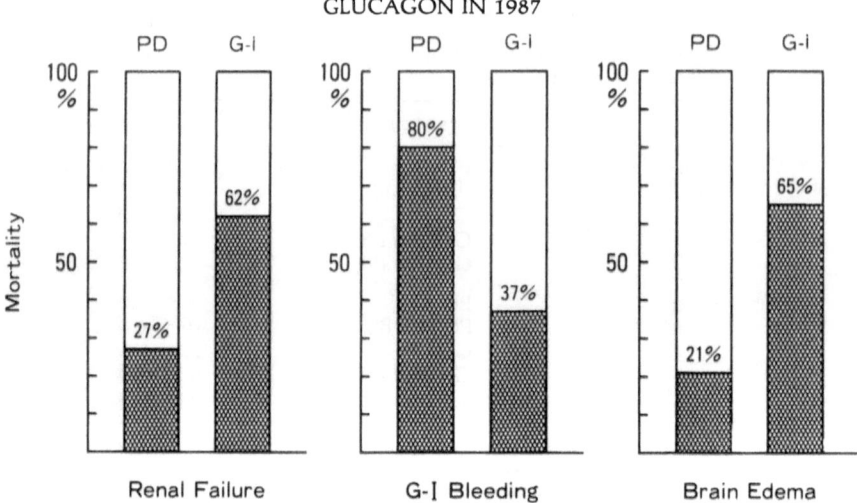

Figure 10.1 Comparison of complication rates among fatal cases from groups of FH patients treated with either prednisolone (PD) or glucagon–insulin (G–I)

Cause of death

It is well-known that several critical complications increase the mortality rate associated with this disease. Therefore, the cause of death was compared between the two therapy groups. Regarding complications such as renal failure, upper gastrointestinal bleeding and brain oedema, the incidence of gastrointestinal bleeding was lower in fatal cases treated with G–I than that in the prednisolone-treated patients. However, renal failure and brain oedema were common fatal complications among the cases who were given G–I (Figure 10.1). The reason for these fatal complications being observed more frequently in this group might be related to the prolonged survival period. Although infections also represent a critical complication in this condition, in our series it was difficult to determine differences in frequency between both groups, since the cases were not always autopsied.

FH THERAPY

It might be true that the introduction of G–I therapy has contributed to improve the survival rate of FH. As shown in Figure 10.2, it can be concluded from our results that the introduction of G–I therapy improved the survival rate particularly in the early critical period of FH. However, as the cause of death shows, therapy for FH should be directed not only to the immediate repair of acute liver failure resulting from massive liver cell necrosis, but also to protect against and improve very critical complications. Table 10.6 shows

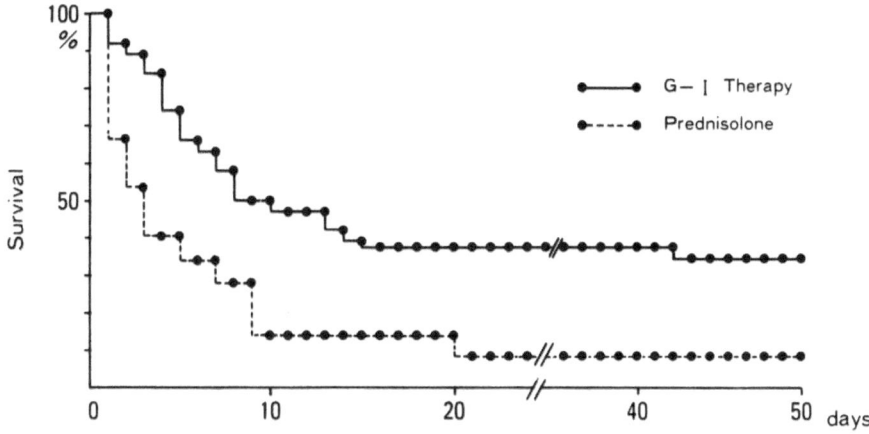

Figure 10.2   Cumulative survival curves for prednisolone (PD) and glucagon–insulin (G–I) treatment groups of FH patients

Table 10.6   Available therapies for fulminant hepatitis

	Therapeutic regimen
Liver cell necrosis	(a) Glucagon–insulin therapy (b) Glucose
Hepatic encephalopathy	(a) Plasmapheresis (b) Branched chain amino-acids (Fischer[13]) (c) Lactulose
Brain oedema	(a) Mannitol, glycerin (b) Head up position (30–45°)
Coagulation	(a) Fresh frozen plasma (b) Antithrombin III
Gastrointestinal bleeding	(a) H_2-receptor antagonist (b) Infusion of secretin
Renal failure	(a) Plasmapheresis (artificial kidney) (b) Diuretic
Infection	(a) Antibiotics

the available current therapies for FH. The following therapeutic modalities have recently been introduced for the treatment of FH: G–I therapy for the stimulation of liver regeneration, as reported here; plasmapheresis and branched chain amino-acids[13] for the improvement of hepatic encephalopathy; mannitol or glycerin and head-up position for the prevention and treatment of brain oedema; administration of antithrombin III for disseminated intravascular

Table 10.7 Survival rates in the different therapy groups of FH patients (Nationwide Survey[16])

Therapy		1982	1983	1984		Total
G–I	(+)	15/59 (25.4%)	20/64 (31.3%)	30/95 (31.6%)		65/218 (29.8%)
	(−)	4/22 (18.2%)	4/21 (19.0%)	3/22 (13.6%)		11/65 (16.9%)
BE	(+)	2/5 (40.0%)	3/6 (50.0%)	2/6 (33.3%)		7/17 (41.1%)
	(−)	17/76 (22.4%)	21/79 (26.5%)	31/111 (27.9%)		69/266 (25.9%)
PP	(+)	15/45 (33.3%)	18/50 (36.0%)	25/84 (29.8%)		58/179 (32.4%)
	(−)	4/36 (11.1%)	6/35 (17.1%)	8/33 (24.2%)		18/104 (17.3%)
SD	(+)	13/58 (22.4%)	13/57 (22.8%)	19/71 (26.8%)		45/186 (24.1%)
	(−)	6/23 (26.1%)	6/22 (27.2%)	14/46 (30.4%)		26/91 (28.5%)

G–I = glucagon–insulin therapy; BE = blood exchange; PP = plasmapheresis; SD = steroid hormone

coagulopathy (DIC); H_2-receptor antagonists for upper gastrointestinal bleeding therapy; dialysis for renal failure; and antibiotics for infection. Therefore, in order to achieve a decrease in mortality rates, patients should be treated in combination with each therapy. However, according to our data, the therapeutic effect of plasmapheresis seems to have been overestimated; in the subacute form of FH the mortality rate of the patients being treated with plasmapheresis never decreased. Therefore, the application of a clinical staging system is absolutely necessary for the selection of a mode of therapy.

CONCLUSION

In conclusion, the usefulness of G–I therapy for FH was evaluated in our Institution. According to our data, G–I therapy either with or without combination with plasmapheresis, contributed to decrease mortality, particularly in the acute form of this disease. Takahashi[16] has evaluated the usefulness of G–I, blood exchange, plasmapheresis, and steroid hormone therapy, based upon a nationwide survey. As shown in Table 10.7, among these therapies, G–I therapy and plasmapheresis may be preferable, but administration of steroid hormones should be discontinued, since there is a lack of difference in survival rate between cases treated with and without these agents. This result may support our conclusion.

The administration of G–I therapy is a very simple procedure and therefore can be performed in every institution. However, it may be advisable to start G–I therapy at an early stage, even when the progression to FH is only suspected in the patient with acute hepatitis. From the results described in this paper, G–I therapy should be considered one of the main therapeutic approaches for FH.

References

1. Sherlock S, Parbhoo P. The management of hepatic failure. *Postgrad Med J* 1971; 47: 493–498.
2. Trey C, Davidson CS. The management of fulminant hepatic failure. In: Popper H, Schaffner F, eds. *Progress in Liver Disease*, 3rd edn. New York: Grune & Stratton, 1970: 282–298.
3. Karvoutzis GG, Redeker AG, Peters RL. Long-term follow-up studies on patients surviving fulminant viral hepatitis. *Gastroenterology* 1974; 67: 870–877.
4. Takahashi Y, Shimizu M, Kosaka M. Nation-wide statistics of fulminant hepatitis (Jap). *Saishin Igaku* 1979; 34: 2285–2292.
5. Bucher NLR, Swaffield MN. Regulation of hepatic regeneration in rats by synergistic action of insulin and glucagon. *Proc Natl Acad Sci USA* 1975; 72: 1157–1160.
6. Starzl TE, Watanabe K, Porter KA, Putnam CW. Effects of insulin, glucagon and insulin/glucagon infusion on liver morphology and liver cell division after complete portacaval shunt in dogs. *Lancet* 1976; 1: 821–825.
7. Caruana JA, Gage AA. Increased uptake of insulin and glucagon by the liver as a signal for regeneration. *Surg Gynecol Obstet* 1980; 150: 390–394.
8. Caruana JA, Goldman JK, Camara DS, Gage AA. Insulin, glucagon and glucose in the regeneration response of the liver. *Surg Gynecol Obstet* 1981; 153: 726–730.
9. Leffert HL, Koch KS, Moran T, Rubalcava B. Hormonal control of rat liver regeneration. *Gastroenterology* 1979; 76: 1470–1482.
10. McGowan JA, Strain AJ, Bucher NLR. DNA synthesis in primary cultures of adult rat hepatocytes in a defined medium: Effect of epidermal growth factor, insulin, glucagon, and cyclic AMP. *J Cell Physiol* 1981; 108: 353–363.
11. Farivar M, Wands JR, Isselbacher KJ, Bucher NLR. Effect of insulin and glucagon on fulminant murine hepatitis. *N Engl J Med* 1976; 296: 1517–1519.
12. Okita K, Noda K, Fukumoto Y, Kodama T, Takemoto T. Protection against liver cell necrosis by synergistic action of glucagon and insulin. *Acta Hepatol Japan* 1978; 19: 848–853.
13. Fischer JE, Baldessarini RJ. False neurotransmitters and hepatic failure. *Lancet* 1971; 2: 75–80.
14. Berk PD, Popper H. Fulminant hepatic failure. *Am J Gastroenterol* 1978; 69: 349–400.
15. Report from the European Association for the Study of the Liver (EASL). Randomized trial of steroid therapy in acute liver failure. *Gut* 1979; 20: 620–623.
16. Takahashi Z. Annual report of nation-wide statistics of fulminant hepatitis – 1982, 1983, 1985. (Supported by a Grant-in-Aid from the Japanese Ministry of Health and Welfare.) Personal communication, 1985.

DISCUSSION

Vilardell   Dr Okita, how did you compare the prednisolone-treated patients with the others? Was this some sort of historical control study?

Okita   This was a prospective uncontrolled study. We chose to compare glucagon/insulin with prednisolone because many doctors in Japan often use prednisolone for the treatment of fulminant hepatitis because they still believe it is effective in such cases. Therefore, we collected prospectively prednisolone-treated cases and glucagon/insulin-treated cases and compared them.

Baker I think it must be a difficult task for you to try to discriminate between the effects of blood exchange and plasmapheresis and prednisolone in combination with glucagon/insulin therapy in order to say which one is really proving beneficial. But one way that it seems to me you might be able to at least approach this would be to know what the control studies in Japan have shown with respect to plasmapheresis and blood exchange therapies. Have such studies been done in Japan? Is there any controlled trial of plasmapheresis for fulminant hepatic failure that has been carried out or a controlled trial of blood exchange, for example?

Okita I understand your point, but unfortunately in Japan we are unable to do such double-blind or single-blind trials with these very severe cases, so all we can do is actually what we have done, which is to compare historical control studies. We cannot do a controlled trial, which of course is quite a different situation from your countries.

Baker From how far back do your historical controls date? For how long have you been collecting cases for your study?

Okita Our study includes cases gathered for 10 years, from 1976 to 1986.

Carr-Locke I am concerned with the fact that several times this afternoon we have reached a point where an ethical question has prevented the evaluation of a trial which obviously requires to be done, and I do not entirely understand why that is so. If you have a clinical situation where you have no 'treatment', which is basically the case with acute fulminant hepatic failure, where we have tried so many things and failed, and you have the possibility of evaluating a new treatment even if you do not know if it will work or not, surely it ought to lend itself to clinical evaluation and not be an ethical problem, because you are offering these patients some new possibility, even if you do not know if it is going to succeed. Why has this continued to be an ethical problem?

Okita I understand what you are saying. Perhaps it depends on a cultural or religious factor rooted in the background of the Japanese people. But the fact remains that in Japan we simply cannot do such trials in this type of very severe cases. It is definitely a question of ethics to us. If, for example, you study H_2-blockers in gastric ulcer cases, this problem does not arise because these patients do not die but, as you know, in cases of fulminant hepatic failure there is a mortality rate of 80 or 90%, which at least according to Japanese standards, makes it a very delicate situation.

Vilardell It would seem to me that the ethical problem would begin with the physician himself, where he might believe that one treatment is superior to another, even if there is no statistical evidence to prove this. But if he has convinced himself, from an ethical point of view, that the therapy he is using works, it will be very difficult to have him use any other. Would you agree with that?

Baker I think you could also approach Dr Carr-Locke's statement in a different way. For all we know, glucagon may be harmful in these very ill patients, but at least if you do a controlled trial you only put 50% of the patients at risk to a harmful effect if there is one, and we have heard quite a few things about complications today. In that connection I wanted to say that you showed some complications but did not mention hypoglycaemia and in these patients you might expect that hypoglycaemia would be much more severe because of their more severe liver disease than in the cases Professor Oka presented.

Okita Actually, in patients receiving glucagon/insulin infusion we monitored carefully the blood sugar levels and in those where they became alarmingly low we treated hypoglycaemia by infusing a 10 or 15% glucose solution in order to prevent severe hypoglycaemia.

Vilardell Yes, Professor Oka showed that hypoglycaemia was more common in his series of acute hepatitis cases than in the other group, and some of his patients had to be withdrawn from the study because of hypoglycaemia symptoms, so indeed, this may be a problem. In my own view, that would certainly justify the carrying out of a controlled clinical trial.

11
A clinical perspective on hepatic regeneration

A. L. BAKER

INTRODUCTION

Despite continuing study, uncertainty persists about the basic mechanisms underlying hepatic regeneration. A growing body of evidence suggests that circulating hormones and other growth promoting factors are involved in the process, but there is less information about how these substances bind to hepatocyte membrane and initiate intracellular signals resulting in DNA synthesis and cell proliferation. The purpose of this review is to summarize recent studies which shed light on some of the processes involved in hepatic regeneration and to highlight the clinical studies which have attempted to apply these principles to the treatment of patients with liver disease.

PROCESSES INVOLVED IN HEPATIC REGENERATION

Hepatic regeneration in animals

At least four peptide hormones – insulin, glucagon, epidermal growth factor and thyroid hormone – along with calcium and some nutrients, particularly amino-acids, appear to be involved in hepatic regeneration (Table 11.1). Supporting evidence for a role for these substances comes from whole animal experiments with confirmation in cell cultures, usually with adult rat hepatocytes which ordinarily do not divide in culture. Early studies demonstrated that portal blood was necessary for maintenance of liver size and the normal regenerative response to hepatic resection. Starzl *et al.*[1] showed that auxiliary

Table 11.1   Circulating regulators of hepatic regeneration in animals

Probably important	Possibly important
Insulin	Corticosteroids
Glucagon	Prostaglandins
Epidermal growth factor	Liver homogenates
Thyroid hormone	Hepatic stimulator substances
Calcium	Glycylhistidyllysine
Nutrients	

homografts in dogs atrophied unless supplied by splanchnic blood. Portacaval transposition in dogs also resulted in hepatic atrophy, excluding the possibility that the quantity of hepatic blood flow was the key factor rather than its content[2]. Additional studies using eviscerated rats and dogs demonstrated that hepatic regeneration after partial hepatectomy was subnormal[3-5]. Insulin and glucagon were both required to return the regenerative response toward normal in rats, whereas insulin alone appeared to be sufficient in dogs; the reason for these species differences is unknown. A number of additional novel experiments, reviewed elsewhere, have provided further evidence that factors contained in portal blood are involved in the control of hepatic regeneration[6,7]. Pharmacological doses of glucagon have generally been required to maximize the regenerative response, whereas physiological doses of insulin are generally sufficient. These studies do not exclude the possibility that additional growth factors are involved in the hepatic regeneration.

Epidermal growth factor is unique among putative hepatic growth factors in that it can induce a significant hepatocyte proliferation in unoperated animals[7,8]. Preliminary studies have suggested that this substance, like insulin, declines after hepatic response, suggesting that hepatocyte uptake might be involved and providing presumptive support for a role in hepatic regeneration[9]. In addition, epidermal growth factor can induce proliferation in adult rat hepatocyte cultures[9]. Like epidermal growth factor, thyroid hormone can produce a significant but small proliferative response when infused into the peripheral veins of unoperated rats[10]. The regenerative response following hepatic resection is impaired in thyroidectomized rats[11]. Thyroid hormone, in conjunction with insulin, glucagon, and amino-acids can enhance the proliferation response in cell culture systems[12]. Parathyroidectomized animals also show a subnormal regenerative response following hepatic resection[13]. This effect can be reversed by the administration of intraperitoneal parathormone or calcium. Calcium is also required for optimal proliferating rat hepatocytes in culture[14]. Likewise, amino-acids contribute to the proliferative response in unoperated animals and in liver cell cultures[8,10].

Another line of evidence provides supportive evidence for the importance of circulating growth factors, particularly insulin and glucagon. Following partial hepatectomy, blood glucagon levels rapidly rise and insulin levels gradually fall, followed in the rat by increased hepatic DNA synthesis at 12–18 h[15–17]. By 24 h, mitoses can be identified in the liver remnant, and the mass of the organ is usually restored within 4–6 days. A metabolic stimulus to change blood hormone levels has been excluded in some studies by documenting normal blood glucose levels during the proliferative response, suggesting that hormonal secretion is involved in liver regeneration[17].

Other potential growth factors

A variety of other substances which may have hepatotrophic effects have received some study, including prostaglandins, corticosteroids, and liver homogenates (Table 11.1)[18–20]. Recently, attention has focussed on several hepatic stimulator substances prepared from the cytosol of regenerating rat livers. LaBrecque[21] has isolated a hepatic stimulator substance which has a molecular weight of approximately 10 000 and can induce DNA synthesis in liver cell cultures and in unoperated rats. This substance is heat stable and its effects are specific to the liver. Francavilla et al.[22] identified two additional hepatic stimulator substances, prepared from regenerating rat fetal liver, with molecular weights of 50 000 and 300 000. When injected into rats two days after the administration of dimethylnitrosamine for the production of fulminant hepatic failure, both substances improved mortality compared to saline-treated controls, although only the high molecular weight hepatic stimulator substance produced a statistically significant effect. The chemical nature of these substances has not yet been clarified, leaving some doubt about the importance of these observations, but further study of these hepatic stimulator substances is certainly warranted.

A circulating tripeptide, glycylhistidyllysine, may be an important growth factor in a number of culture systems[23,24]. This tripeptide binds iron and copper and can interact with hepatocyte membranes in vitro, contributing to hepatocyte adherence to culture plates and cell proliferation. Serum is ordinarily required for hepatocyte adherence and growth in cultures, and glycylhistidyllysine may be an important serum component which initiates this response. Additional studies are needed to determine whether this tripeptide is important in liver regeneration in vivo.

Interaction of hepatotrophic factors

Evidence that growth factors interact in a precise pattern to initiate cell proliferation has been recently reviewed by Leffert et al.[9] and Armato and Andreis[18]. These workers have suggested that some factors, commitment factors or mitogen activators, initiate cell proliferation and include epidermal growth factor, nutrients, and perhaps prostaglandins and hepatic stimulator substance. Other growth factors serve as intracyclic regulators, potentiating the proliferative response, and include epidermal growth factor, insulin, glucagon, and perhaps calcium. After adult rat hepatocytes are established in culture, a medium change, supplying ionic constituents and nutrients, or insulin and glucagon with a medium change, stimulate little DNA synthesis. When the medium is changed and epidermal growth factor is added from 0–12 h, DNA synthesis occurs; the effect is retained even if epidermal growth factor is removed between 3 and 6 h, if insulin and glucagon are subsequently added. Insulin and glucagon need not be added for up to 10 h but must be present for at least 6 h to produce a maximal growth response. Such observations suggest that epidermal growth factor may initiate hepatocyte proliferation which is subsequently potentiated by insulin and glucagon. Because of the presence of non-parenchymal hepatic cells in these cultures, additional hormones and mediators may also be involved. Such observations underscore the complexity of liver cell growth and suggest that the process is under careful biological control.

Binding of circulating growth factors to hepatocytes

Whatever the precise relationship among circulating hepatotrophic factors, these substances are generally thought to bind to hepatocyte membranes to initiate intracellular signals resulting in hepatic DNA synthesis and cell proliferation. Indirect effects are also possible, perhaps through peripheral nutritional or hormonal influences or by effect on non-parenchymal hepatic cells to promote matrix formation.

Previous studies have shown that insulin and glucagon extraction are increased across the liver in the immediate post-hepatectomy state[25]. More recent studies demonstrated that insulin and glucagon levels increased following limited (42%) and extended (72%) partial hepatectomy in dogs, whereas the metabolic clearance rate and $t_{1/2}$ for insulin and glucagon were unchanged[17]. Serum glucose remained normal, indicating that there was no metabolic stimulus to hormone secretion. These results, plus the observation that insulin/C-peptide molar ratios were unchanged following partial hepatectomy suggested that the raised hormone levels were due to increased secretion, compatible with a role in hepatic regeneration. Direct assays of hepatocyte plasma membrane insulin and glucagon binding, however, have provided conflicting results, both following partial hepatectomy and carbon tetrachloride hepatotoxicity[26,27].

Epidermal growth factor (EGF) binding to hepatocyte plasma membranes is also uncertain. Some investigators have reported a fall in EGF levels following partial hepatectomy, consistent with increased uptake. Measurements have been hampered by the presence of an EGF propeptide in many of the tissues to which EGF may bind, however[28].

Intracellular signals initiating hepatocyte proliferation

Although the interaction between circulating growth factors and the hepatocyte membrane needs further study, a growing body of literature refers to the intracellular signals which initiate hepatic regeneration. Both the insulin and EGF receptors have tyrosine kinase activity, as do the oncogene products of acutely transforming retroviruses[28]. This observation suggests one possible mechanism by which circulating growth factors may initiate cell replication.

Specific mRNAs may initiate DNA synthesis and cell division[29-31]. Present evidence suggests that following partial hepatectomy liver mRNA abundance increases, without any obvious change in the spectrum of gene products. This change is in marked contrast to that which is observed in the maturing fetal liver, where the spectrum of mRNAs is markedly different from that in adults[32]. It has been generally assumed that liver cells retrogress before division following partial hepatectomy, but α-fetoprotein mRNA content does not show a disproportionate increase. A recent study using carbon tetrachloride hepatotoxicity as a model for hepatic regeneration did demonstrate a specific increase in α-fetoprotein mRNA content[33]. Some RNA transcripts, such as those controlling enzymes of the urea cycle which are increased following partial hepatectomy, doubtless represent metabolic adaptation and the need to maintain the animal's viability, rather than to participate in cell replication. At least two oncogenes, *ras* and *myc*, increase during liver regeneration at the time of maximum DNA synthesis[31,34]. Additional study will be required to determine whether proteins synthesized by these genes control DNA synthesis following partial hepatectomy.

Yet another area for further study is the recent evidence that an unusual purine nucleotide, di-adenosine $5',5''''-P_1,P_4$-tetraphosphate (AP_4A) is increased in hepatocytes following hepatic resection but before DNA replication occurs[35,36]. AP_4A may stimulate DNA synthesis through DNA polymerase. This nucleotide is found in the circulation but cannot cross the normal plasma membrane; altered permeability and intracellular accumulation might result from the binding of this circulating growth factor.

CLINICAL TRIALS OF HEPATOTROPHIC FACTORS IN HUMAN LIVER DISEASE

Hepatic regeneration in humans

The basic hypothesis underlying the use of insulin and glucagon in clinical trials is that these hormones are hepatotrophic in humans, as appears to be the case in experimental animals. Direct proof of this assumption is lacking. However, it seems reasonable to believe that such a basic biological process is under similar control among mammalian species. In addition, two lines of indirect evidence suggest that factors contained in splanchnic blood are probably hepatotrophic in humans. First, hepatic atrophy is a predictable result of total portacaval shunting, but is a less frequent complication of the distal splenorenal shunt[37,38], where portal blood flow is maintained. Second, the pattern of serum hormones, particularly insulin and glucagon, following partial hepatectomy is similar to that in experimental animals; peak levels of glucagon and the decline in insulin precede hepatic regeneration, suggesting that these hormones may be important in regulating the process.

Controlled trials of insulin and glucagon for the treatment of liver disease

In 1981 we reported the results of a randomized controlled trial of 50 patients using insulin and glucagon for severe alcoholic hepatitis[39]. This study showed no overall improvement in mortality in the treated patients, but in study subjects with the most severe hepatic disease, prothrombin time greater than 3 s prolonged, there was a trend toward improved survival ($p < 0.10$). The absolute decrease in the total serum bilirubin and prothrombin time were greater in the treated patients. We have now studied an additional 22 patients according to the same protocol. All patients gave informed written consent to the study. For entry into the study, patients were required to have a history of heavy, daily alcohol consumption for at least a year (80 g or more daily), repetitive binge drinking for years, or family substantiation of heavy alcohol consumption for years without specific quantitation. The diagnosis of alcoholic hepatitis was established by the presence of abnormal liver chemistry tests, with the aspartate aminotransferase (AST) more markedly elevated than the alanine aminotransferase (ALT); a liver biopsy was required if the prothrombin time was less than 3 s prolonged and the platelet count greater than 60 000, making the procedure reasonably safe. Patients were randomized by sealed envelope to receive insulin (2 U h^{-1}) and glucagon (200 μg h^{-1}) in 200 ml of 5% dextrose in water by a peripheral or central vein for 12 h daily for 3 weeks. Human serum albumin was added to the bottles containing hormones to prevent adsorption to the infusion apparatus and to the control bottles to maintain an identical appearance. Clinical status was assessed daily, and liver chemistry tests were measured and the results recorded three times weekly. During the first few days of treatment, patients were monitored by frequent measurements of blood glucose on venous blood specimens or by Dextrostix, and additional glucose was infused as needed to prevent hypoglycaemia.

There were six deaths in the insulin and glucagon-treated group and nine

Table 11.2   Mortality in insulin and glucagon-treated and control patients

	Insulin and glucagon	Control
Total no. of patients studied	35	37
Total no. of deaths	6	9
No. of patients with prothrombin time >3 s prolonged	21	22
Deaths in patients with prothrombin time >3 s prolonged	2	7*

In comparison with controls, *$p < 0.10$, other differences also not significant

Table 11.3   Liver biochemical tests in insulin and glucagon-treated and control patients

Test	Baseline value	After 3 weeks	Absolute change	p-value
Serum bilirubin (mg dl^{-1})				
Insulin and glucagon	9.8 ± 1.3	4.2 ± 1.1	-5.1 ± 1.2	<0.05
Control	12.1 ± 1.3	10.6 ± 1.0	-1.6 ± 1.3	
Prothrombin time (s)				
Insulin and glucagon	16.1 ± 0.4	14.1 ± 0.3	-2.3 ± 0.2	<0.05
Control	16.5 ± 0.5	15.9 ± 1.0	-0.4 ± 0.3	
Aspartate aminotransferase (IU)				
Insulin and glucagon	101 ± 14	90 ± 16	-14 ± 15	NS
Control	125 ± 5	91 ± 14	-38 ± 14	
Alkaline phosphatase (IU)				
Insulin and glucagon	100 ± 9	87 ± 13	-13 ± 8	NS
Control	99 ± 10	82 ± 5	-14 ± 6	
Albumin (g dl^{-1})				
Insulin and glucagon	2.5 ± 0.2	2.8 ± 0.2	0.4 ± 0.2	NS
Control	2.5 ± 0.2	2.9 ± 0.1	0.5 ± 0.2	

in the control group, a difference which was not statistically significant (Table 11.2). As in the initial study, the combined results in 72 patients showed a trend toward improved survival in the patients with the most severe disease, prothrombin time greater than 3 s prolonged at entry, but the results again failed to achieve statistical significance ($p < 0.10$) (Table 11.2). The absolute change in total serum bilirubin and prothrombin time were significant (Table 11.3). The other clinical and biochemical measurements carried out in this study did not change significantly. These results suggested that insulin and glucagon might be beneficial for the most severely ill patients with alcoholic hepatitis, but studies at the University of Chicago have not yet confirmed this possibility.

An additional study in 84 patients, using a similar protocol at the University of Southern California, has also been completed. No beneficial effect on survival or liver function could be found[40]. Recently, an additional trial, this one a multicentre investigation from Hungary, has been completed, and the results are discussed elsewhere in this volume. In this trial insulin and glucagon were infused over 4–6 h three times daily for 3 weeks, and a significant improvement in mortality was observed in the treated patients. Taken together, these studies suggest that further investigation of insulin and glucagon therapy for alcoholic hepatitis is warranted. While the precise mechanism of any beneficial effect in humans is uncertain, the results from the Hungarian study suggest that short, repeated doses of insulin and glucagon may be more beneficial than the longer infusions used in the American studies.

Japanese investigators became interested in the use of insulin and glucagon for the treatment of fulminant hepatic failure, because of the frequency of this life-threatening illness in Japan, and the experimental and human clinical data suggest that these hormones might provide an effective treatment. This illness might be more responsive to treatment by hepatotrophic factors than alcoholic hepatitis, since hepatocellular necrosis is the major histologic feature of the early phase of the illness. Oka et al. reported uncontrolled observations using this treatment in 64 patients from several Japanese medical centres and compared the results to a national survey of fulminant hepatic failure in Japan that predated the use of insulin and glucagon[41,42]. Of the 64 patients receiving insulin and glucagon, 29 (45%) recovered, compared with a survival of 19% reported in the national survey. Insulin and glucagon were administered usually in doses of 10 units and 1 mg respectively over 2–6 h in a solution of dextrose in water. Some patients received two or three infusions daily, but the total period of treatment varied widely. Additional treatments, including exchange transfusions, fresh frozen plasma, and corticosteroids were often administered in addition to insulin and glucagon. Based on these results, a multicentre controlled study was begun several years ago, and the results are reported in detail elsewhere in this volume. The selection criteria excluded the patients with the most severe hepatic failure and the most markedly prolonged prothrombin times, so that the study patients had a relatively low risk for mortality. No improvement was noted in survival in the insulin and glucagon-treated patients compared with the controls, but there was a more rapid improvement in the total serum bilirubin and the prothrombin time in the treated patients. Here again, as with alcoholic hepatitis, additional controlled studies seem warranted. Inclusion of patients with the most severe fulminant hepatic failure is justified, particularly because hypoglycaemia and other complications could outweigh any beneficial effects of the treatment on mortality[39].

Future developments

Additional understanding of the basic mechanisms underlying hepatic regeneration should lead to valuable clinical applications. Better ways to assess the degree of hepatic damage and monitor hepatic regeneration should permit the identification of the patients who can benefit most from new approaches to treatment. Additional understanding of the intracellular signals which initiate DNA synthesis and cell replication may open new options for the treatment of human hepatic disease.

Additional clinical trials need not await a full understanding of the mechanisms underlying hepatic regeneration, particularly considering the life-threatening nature of many human liver diseases and the lack of effective treatment. As pointed out in a previous review[6], future studies should adhere to several basic principles. First, only randomized controlled trials can provide objective evidence of a beneficial effect of new therapeutic approaches. Second, mortality should only be used as the key endpoint to be sought in most liver diseases, particularly those with a high mortality such as alcoholic hepatitis and fulminant hepatic failure. Third, trials need to be designed to search for possible complications of therapy, such as hypoglycaemia when insulin is part of the therapeutic regimen. Future exciting developments in this field are anticipated.

Acknowledgement

This work was supported in part by a grant from the Fairbairn Trust Fund and the Liver Research Fund.

References

1. Marchioro T L, Porter K A, Dickinson T C, Faris T D, Starzl T E. Physiologic requirements for auxiliary liver transplantation. *Surg Gynecol Obstet* 1965; 121: 17–31.
2. Starzl T E, Francavilla A, Halgrimson C G, Francavilla F R, Porter K A, Brown T H, Putnam C W. The origin, hormonal nature, and action of hepatotrophic substances in portal venous blood. *Surg Gynecol Obstet* 1973; 137: 179–199.
3. Max M H, Price J B, Takeshige K, Voorhees A B. The role of factors of portal origin in modifying hepatic regeneration. *J Surg Res* 1972; 12: 120–123.
4. Bucher N L R, Swaffield M N. Regulation of hepatic regeneration in rats by synergistic action of insulin and glucagon. *Proc Natl Acad Sci USA* 1975; 72: 1157–1160.
5. Starzl T E, Francavilla A, Porter K A, Benichom J. The effect upon the liver of evisceration with or without hormone replacement. *Surg Gynecol Obstet* 1978; 146: 524–531.
6. Baker A L. Hepatotrophic factors: basic concepts and clinical implications. *Acta Med Scand* 1985; Suppl 703: 201–208.
7. Bucher N L R, Patel U, Cohen S. Hormonal factors and liver growth. *Adv Enz Regul* 1978; 16: 205–213.
8. Bucher N L R, Patel U, Cohen S. Hormonal factors concerned with liver regeneration. In: Porter R, Whelan J, eds. *Hepatotrophic Factors*. Ciba Foundation Symposium, No. 55. Amsterdam: Elsevier, Excerpta Medica, North-Holland, 1978: 95–107.

9. Leffert H L, Koch K S, Moran T, Rubalcava B. Hormonal control of rat liver regeneration. *Gastroenterology* 1979; 76: 1470–1482.
10. Short J, Brown R F, Husakova A, Gilbertson J R, Zemel R, Lieberman I. Induction of deoxyribonucleic acid synthesis in the liver of the intact animal. *J Biol Chem* 1972; 247: 1757–1766.
11. Canzanelli A D, Rapport D, Guild P. Control of liver regeneration and nucleic acid content by the thyroid with observation on the effects of pyrimidines. *Am J Physiol* 1949; 157: 225–233.
12. Leffert H L, Koch K S. Proliferation of hepatocytes. In: Porter R, Whelan J, eds. *Hepatotrophic Factors.* Ciba Foundation Symposium, No. 55. Amsterdam: Elsevier, Excerpta Medica, North-Holland, 1978: 61–94.
13. Rixon R H, Whitfield J F. The control of liver regeneration by parathyroid hormone and calcium. *J Cell Physiol* 1976; 87: 147–156.
14. Andreis P G, Armato U, Whitfield J F. The calcium-dependent stimulation of the proliferation of neonatal rat hepatocytes by imidazole and indomethacin. *Chem-Biol Interact* 1981; 37: 25–39.
15. Leffert H L, Alexander N M, Faloona G, Rubalcava B, Unger R H. Specific endocrine and hormonal receptor changes associated with liver regeneration in adult rats. *Proc Natl Acad Sci USA* 1975; 72: 4033–4036.
16. Morley C G D, Kuku S, Rubenstein A H, Boyer J L. Serum hormone levels following partial hepatectomy in the rat. *Biochem Biophys Res Commun* 1975; 67: 653–661.
17. Cohen D M, Jaspan J B, Polonsky K S, Lever E G, Moossa A R. Pancreatic hormone profiles and metabolism post-hepatectomy in the dog. Evidence for a hepatotrophic role of insulin, glucagon, and pancreatic polypeptide. *Gastroenterology* 1984; 87: 679–687.
18. Armato U, Andreis P G. Prostaglandins of the F series are extremely powerful growth factors in primary neonatal rat hepatocytes. *Life Sci* 1983; 33: 1745–1755.
19. Miura Y, Fukui N. Prostaglandins as possible triggers for liver regeneration after partial hepatectomy. A review. *Cell Mol Biol* 1979; 25: 179–184.
20. Blomqvist K. Growth stimulation in the liver and tumor development following intraperitoneal injections of liver homogenates in the rat. *Acta Pathol Microbiol Scand* 1957; Suppl 121: 65–87.
21. LaBrecque D R, Bachur N R. Hepatic stimulator substance: physicochemical characteristics and specificity. *Am J Physiol* 1982; 242: G281–G288.
22. Francavilla A, DiLeo A, Polimeno L, Gavaler J, Pellicci R, Todo S, Kam I, Prelich J, Makowka L, Starzl T E. The effect of hepatic stimulatory substance, isolated from regenerating hepatic cytosol, and 50 000 and 300 000 subfractions in enhancing survival in experimental acute hepatic failure in rats treated with D-galactosamine. *Hepatology* 1986; 6: 1346–1351.
23. Pickart L, Thaler M M. Tripeptide in human serum which prolongs survival of normal liver cells and stimulates the growth of hepatoma cells. *Nature New Biol* 1973; 243: 85–87.
24. Pickart L, Thaler M M. Growth-modulating tripeptide (glycylhistidyllysine): association with copper and iron in plasma, and stimulation of adhesiveness and growth of hepatoma cells in culture by tripeptide–metal ion complexes. *J Cell Physiol* 1980; 102: 129–139.
25. Caruana J A, Gage A A. Increased uptake of insulin and glucagon as a signal of regeneration. *Surg Gynecol Obstet* 1980; 150: 390–394.
26. Mourelle M, Rubalcava B. Changes in the insulin and glucagon receptors in the regenerating liver following intoxication with carbon tetrachloride. *Biochem Biophys Res Commun* 1979; 88: 189–198.
27. Pezzino V, Vigneri R, Cohen D, Goldfine I D. Regenerating rat liver: insulin and glucagon serum levels and receptor binding. *Endocrinology* 1981; 108: 2163–2169
28. Editorial. Polypeptide growth factors: a clinical perspective. *Lancet* 1985, 2: 251–253.
29. Friedman J M, Chung E Y, Darnell J E Jr. Gene expression during liver regeneration. *J Mol Biol* 1984; 179: 37–53.
30. Petropoulos C, Andrews G, Tamaoki T, Fausto N. α-Fetoprotein and albumin mRNA levels in liver regeneration and carcinogenesis. *J Biol Chem* 1983; 258: 4901–4906.
31. Fausto N. Messenger RNA in regenerating liver: implications for the understanding of regulated growth. *Mol Cell Biochem* 1984; 59: 131–147.

32. Andrews G K, Dziadek M, Tamaoki T. Expression and methylation of the mouse α-fetoprotein gene in embryonic, adult, and neoplastic tissues. *J Biol Chem* 1982; 257: 5148–5153.
33. Panduro A, Shalaby F, Weiner F R, Biempica L, Zern M A, Shafritz D A. Transcriptional switch from albumin to α-fetoprotein and changes in transcription of other genes during carbon tetrachloride-induced liver regeneration. *Biochemistry* 1986; 25: 1414–1420.
34. Goyette M, Petropoulos C J, Shank P R, Fausto N. Expression of a cellular oncogene during liver regeneration. *Science* 1983; 219: 510–512.
35. Yamaguchi N, Kodama M, Ueda K. Di-adenosine tetraphosphate as a signal molecule linked with the functional state of rat liver. *Gastroenterology* 1985; 89: 723–731.
36. Bissell D M. Peculiar purine nucleotide and liver regeneration. *Gastroenterology* 1985; 89: 914–916.
37. Rikkers L F, Rudman D, Galambos J T, Fulenwider T, Millikan W T, Kutner M, Smith R B, Salamn A A, Jones A J, Warren W D. A randomized, controlled trial of the distal splenorenal shunt. *Ann Surg* 1978; 188: 271–281.
38. Yamaoka Y, Sato M, Kimura K, Takasan H, Ozawa K. Role of portal venous blood supply from the pancreas in maintaining hepatic functional reserve. Appraisal of Warren's shunt operation. *Arch Surg* 1978; 113: 981–985.
39. Baker A L, Jaspan J B, Haines N W, Hatfield G E, Krager P S, Schneider J F, The University of Chicago Medical House-Staff. A randomized clinical trial of insulin and glucagon infusion for treatment of alcoholic hepatitis: progress report in 50 patients. *Gastroenterology* 1981; 80: 1410–1414.
40. Radvan G, Kanel G, Redeker A. Insulin and glucagon infusion in acute alcoholic hepatitis. *Gastroenterology* 1982; 82: 1154.
41. Oka H, Okita K, Fujiwara K. Glucagon and insulin therapy in fulminant hepatic failure in Japan. In: Picazo J, ed. *Glucagon in Gastroenterology and Hepatology.* Lancaster: MTP Press, 1982: 171–180.
42. Takahashi Y, Shimizu M, Kosaka M. Nationwide statistics of severe hepatitis (fulminant hepatitis) (Jap). *Saishin Igaku* 1979; 34: 2285–2292.

DISCUSSION

Nikolov   You mentioned several growth factors, but you did not mention fibroplast growth factor or platelet growth factor and I would like to know your opinion about that. On the other hand, I would also like to ask you whether it makes a difference to study liver regeneration in subtotally hepatectomized rats or in toxically-induced liver damage. It has long been known that one tenth of the liver is sufficient to keep all liver functions working, so I find that perhaps it is not the same to do studies in hepatectomized rats or in toxically-induced liver necrosis. Could you please comment on this?

Baker   I certainly agree with your latter point that to study rats or any other experimental animal undergoing partial hepatectomy is an artificial system, as far as what we would like to apply in patients is concerned, and in that sense the kind of study that Dr Fujiwara talked about with a toxically-induced hepatitis in animals is a more realistic kind of study. I presented these studies in partial hepatectomy simply to try to indicate as background material what some of the ideas involved in hepatic regeneration are. If you are asking the question with that aim, then I do think it is worth looking at an artificial system like hepatectomy, at least as far as human disease is concerned, because that way you get rid of many additional factors that may be caused in your model if, for instance, you produce a viral hepatitis in an animal or you give galactosamine, where you would get quite an amount of fat accumulation in the liver. In some sense I think you can look in a purer fashion at what these hepatotrophic substances are doing. But I do agree with your basic point that it is more realistic to look at disease models than it is to look at hepatectomy. With respect to your first comment, I would agree with those first two growth factors that you mentioned. Certainly in a brief talk like this I could not begin to cover all the growth factors that might be mentioned but, indeed, there is evidence that both fibroblast growth factor and platelet-derived growth factor may have effects on hepatocytes. And another area that I did not touch at all, and that I think we are going to hear more about in the next few years, is the role of matrix in the liver, the necessity of the liver to lay down matrix proteins, collagens and other proteins for the liver to grow or to regenerate on, and platelet-derived growth factor and fibroblast growth factor might have effects along those lines which could be equally important to anything going on in the hepatocyte itself, at least in the way we have thought about it up to now.

Fehér I enjoyed your lecture very much Dr Baker, especially your suggestions concerning future studies, and I fully agree with your conclusions. In a new therapeutic modality it is necessary firstly to have a very exact prospective multicentric study; it was the first conclusion of your study and I agree with it totally, and the second conclusion you made is a very important point for us concerning the future because there are three or four multicentre studies going with glucagon/insulin treatment, and I also am of the opinion that the key is the mortality rate. But, unfortunately, in the studies we do, when we reach the point where the difference in the mortality rate is significant between the control and the therapy groups, we must stop the study, because due to an ethical factor we are not allowed to continue. That is why I think that you have shown me a very interesting and convenient way of proceeding with our study in the future.

Vilardell Where do we go from here Dr Baker? Because if I interpret your findings correctly, by carefully stratifying the patients in your study according to those who have the severest liver disease, it seems that you have almost reached significance. That is what it seems to me that you have been showing: low prothrombin times as a parameter of severe disease which has almost led you to reach a significance. If you take mortality as a single parameter, of course, you may find yourself stuck, as anybody else would be, with the fact that you probably need quite a number of patients if you want enough statistical power and you may be unable to do that absolutely on your own. You will probably need a very large study with a great number of patients for that, and actually that is what everybody else is doing. The second problem I can identify here is the differences in technique. You are using therapy in a different way from Professor Fehér, which may also have some bearing on the results. So, what would you suggest now? Would you stop your trial or would you go on? Or would you try to set up a multicentre trial using Professor Fehér's technique?

Baker   Well, it is a difficult thing, but I think that during the time since we began this trial up to now we have learned a good bit about the requirements for a well-designed therapeutic trial. We thought this one was quite good when we started out, but I can tell you now that since then we have learned a great deal about how it could be better. Let me give you some of the ideas that I think ought to go into future designs. Number one is to include the patients who are at risk of death, and number two is that you must include as far as possible the patients who will respond to your therapy. Number one means that you have to identify the patients who are significantly ill with a disease, because if you have in your study a large number of patients who are not seriously ill and therefore are not at risk of death, this fact is going to obscure the benefit that you have for the more severely ill patients. And this, I suspect, has been one of the troubles with our trial, because initially we took all-comers with alcoholic hepatitis with or without associated cirrhosis as long as there was a biopsy or compatible liver chemistry tests and a coagulopathy that prevented diagnosis. In retrospect, we have a few patients in this study who have a quite pure cirrhosis alone, and it is not likely that they are going to respond very well to insulin and glucagon, so that is the second problem that we have at least with two or three patients. We have some patients who were not likely to respond to begin with. So I think those are the two key factors with respect to the patients. Number one, they must be severe enough cases for you to see a difference between your control group and your insulin and glucagon-treated patients. Number two, they must be able to respond to whatever treatment you give, which means that your diagnostic criteria have to exclude those who will not respond, as for example pure cirrhotics or patients with diseases other than alcoholic hepatitis. Then, perhaps, number three could be the details of the therapy. I think that with Professor Fehér's study and with what we heard from Professor Lefèbvre about pulsatile glucagon and insulin secretion, it would at least make sense to give short repeated infusions of insulin and glucagon rather than prolonged infusions such as we gave in our study, but we just happened to choose that because that is what Starlz had done (Starlz T E, Francavilla A, Porter K A, et al. Surg Gynecol Obstet 1978; 146: 524–531).

In the studies that I quoted to you where he did partial portacaval transposition in dogs, he gave continuous infusions for a 12 h period, it seemed to work and there were no previous studies, so we used that approach when we started our trial.

Vilardell   Dr Baker, would you in any way exclude patients with portal hypertension? Because if glucagon increases splanchnic blood flow, I think perhaps this might disturb you when working with this sort of patient.

Baker   I think that the question that you raised earlier is a very interesting one. Of course, patients with alcoholic hepatitis already have a high hepatic blood flow and I wonder if glucagon has the capacity to increase that hepatic blood flow any further. Certainly, in our study we looked for complications of increased bleeding and found none; clinically we did not seem to exacerbate bleeding in these patients. It is an interesting point and it is something that ought to be looked at, but because these patients already have a high liver blood flow as a characteristic of their disease, it would not necessarily make me discard glucagon as part of an effective therapeutic regimen.

General Discussion

Oriol-Bosch   To start this final General Discussion on the great amount of information that has been laid out today, I would like to recall briefly that we began with a review of the effects and mechanisms of action of glucagon. Particularly concerning the effects, I would like to say that these were not only physiological, they were, in the main, pharmacological. We owe to Professor Lefèbvre an outstanding contribution on 'the review of the art'. Then we had two wonderful presentations about upper and lower gastrointestinal radiology by Drs Maruyama and Skucas. Dr Carr-Locke presented us with beautiful data about the dynamics of the biliary tract and the effect of glucagon on the Oddi sphincter which I think was very enlightening. Afterwards, Professor Takemoto showed us very nicely the usefulness of glucagon for endoscopy; his presentation closed the morning session. I should say that the morning General Discussion demonstrated the need for more basic physiological knowledge about secretion patterns and the receptor changes that may occur in order eventually to substantiate the pharmacological views of this natural hormone. In the afternoon we had Dr Fujiwara who presented his experimental studies with the use of combined glucagon and insulin for liver regeneration in the rat which was of great interest. Professor Fehér has thrown some new light on the effectiveness of the treatment of alcoholic hepatitis patients from a multicentre trial. Then Professor Oka showed us the results obtained in a multicentric double-blind study which was optimistic about the effectiveness of glucagon/insulin in acute hepatic failure, while Dr Okita has shown that by combining glucagon/insulin therapy with plasmapheresis and blood exchange in fulminant hepatitis, the survival rate of these patients improves and that, even though the mortality is still high, the results have proved to be much better than those seen with corticosteroids which do not seem to be of great help. Finally, Dr Baker has given us a magnificent lecture which opens new hopes for meeting again in the future because there are still many things to be done with glucagon. On the whole, I should say, these contributions have been enriching for all of us. Now I think we could enter into a General Discussion of all that has been said today and perhaps concentrate on what we might consider as established for glucagon and what still remains to be done.

Vilardell   Yes, perhaps we could try to decide among us where the future lies for glucagon and it might be a good idea to start by reviewing the gastrointestinal tract and see where we think that glucagon has some speculative or real interest. Let us start with the oesophagus. Does anyone think that at this moment glucagon is helping in any way with oesophageal conditions? If so, in which and how?

Carr-Locke   This subject has been brought up in discussion already to a small extent today. I think that where it will not have a place is in any pathological process involving the lower oesophageal sphincter, because glucagon does not seem to play any part in modifying that. However, there are clinical conditions that involve the body of the oesophagus, which we have touched on today, such as diffuse oesophageal spasm, and one of the clinical areas that we still find very difficult is where we have to distinguish patients who come into hospital with chest pain of non-cardiac origin, from those who have cardiac pain. Nitrates are still the most commonly used agents for relieving cardiac pain and they, of course, relieve the pain of smooth muscle spasm too. Now with glucagon we ought to be able to distinguish these. It occurred to me just now that this may be the basis for a certain investigation but whether or not it ought to be a trial I do not know. Perhaps glucagon might have an effect in relieving oesophageal pain without effect in cardiac pain. That is a thought. I think, other than that, it does not seem to be very helpful in the oesophagus.

Vilardell   I would agree with you that this does deserve some attention. Now perhaps we could move on to the stomach, stomach radiology. From what we have heard, the opinion seems to be that the main difficulty lies in the lack of action of glucagon in inhibiting gastric secretion, which leads to preferential use of anticholinergics. Since our Japanese colleagues are the masters of gastric radiology, we should ask them whether they agree with that statement. Dr Maruyama, you mentioned the possibility of using glucagon after an anticholinergic ...

Maruyama Yes. In my opinion and according to my experience, that would be the most sensible way to use glucagon, as I already pointed out before.

Vilardell So you find that there is a limited usefulness for glucagon in gastric radiology. Would it have any other use in the United States, Dr Skucas, or is that also the case there concerning the use of glucagon in gastric radiology?

Skucas I should not say as far as the future, since the camp for glucagon is already now divided in two halves, those who claim that it does help and those who claim that it is just an extra injection where you waste a little extra time and it does not do anything. Those who claim it helps say that by paralysing the stomach barium is prevented from flowing out into the duodenum and obscuring part of the stomach, which is reasonable, but my answer to that argument is to do the examination a little faster so that this does not happen. But basically, there is no answer to that.

Vilardell Well then, let us go on to a different topic. The next subject discussed was the use of glucagon in the colon and in colon radiology and colonoscopy. Are there any further comments?

Carr-Locke Before going any further. I must say that we have bypassed the duodenum slightly here, and I would like to comment on something I did not have time to mention before and which I think nobody else has either. The technique of hypotonic duodenography has really gone out of fashion since endoscopy has been able to take its place, but it is still practised in some areas, and I think glucagon really has a central part to play in paralysing the duodenum for radiographic duodenography.

Skucas I would also like to back-track a little bit because I am afraid that we have also jumped over a very important structure, namely the small bowel. We did not discuss the small bowel at all. I was asked to limit my presentation here to the colon, but nonetheless there is a definite role for glucagon in small bowel radiology that I would like to point out, the so-called enteroclisis, the tube study of the small bowel. In general, once the small bowel is opacified, be it single-contrast or double-contrast, many people do give glucagon to paralyse the small bowel. The main purpose for this is that one can then freely take the appropriate films, turn the patient in whatever position is best and so on. Likewise, when doing enteroclisis, if a lesion is seen, by giving glucagon we paralyse the gut and are able to study the abnormal segment at leisure. Although I am not aware of any study comparing enteroclisis with and without glucagon, as far as accuracy of diagnosis is concerned, most people feel that it is beneficial in enteroclisis.

Vilardell I apologize for having omitted the duodenum and small bowel. Which would be the most important indications in small bowel radiology? What sort of lesions? perhaps tumours or Crohn's disease? Would it not obscure things in the case of malabsorption for instance?

Skucas   It will be primarily in localized focal lesions, be it tumours or Crohn's disease. In obstruction or malabsorption I have not found glucagon of much use. In obstruction, even the need for enteroclisis can be questioned because the bowel is already dilated and one is able to see what is happening in it without the need of additional hypotonia.

Vilardell   If there is nothing more to add about duodenum and small bowel I think we can now proceed with the colon concerning the usefulness of glucagon. Do we all agree that glucagon is useful in colonoscopy and colonic radiology?

Takemoto   Well, as I have already commented before, I think we can definitely agree that glucagon has proved to be sufficiently effective and useful as premedication for colonoscopy and barium enema examinations.

Vilardell   Then we are going to move on to the biliary tract and see what is going on there. What use do we have for glucagon in this area? Should we perhaps use it in biliary colic therapy?

Carr-Locke   During endoscopic procedures in the duodenum we use glucagon to paralyse it for a short period of time, usually for endoscopic retrograde cholangiography (ERCP). Now as far as the therapeutic role, I think we still do not know the full answer to this. There are a number of anecdotal reports of the use of glucagon, in other words, open studies without proper assessment in the literature. There are very few controlled studies and they are usually comparisons with other agents such as anticholinergics and there does not seem to be very much difference between glucagon and the standard anticholinergics and an analgesic like diclofenac (see references 57–61 in Chapter 6 by D. L. Carr-Locke in this book). It seems to be effective when it is assessed in that way, but it is very difficult to do a complete double-blind study in such a situation, and I am sure we all know the difficulties of doing that. On an open basis it does seem to relieve biliary pain and I have used it in that situation.

Vilardell   What about the choleretic effect of glucagon and bile flow? I found what you mentioned this morning was quite exciting.

Carr-Locke   The question of the choleretic effect of glucagon is interesting and I think that is the most recently recognized biliary effect that we know in man. I have already mentioned the place it might have in terms of creating increased bile flow in clinical situations and again I think that this is something that must be looked into. Today I just mentioned a few clinical situations where the use of glucagon in this context could be helpful and I am sure others could think of additional indications where the choleretic effect of glucagon could be useful.

Vilardell   And this calls for future work for sure. Now we are approaching one of the main subjects which is the liver, and I would like the speakers on this subject to comment or add anything which they might think has been left out and to tell us where the future lies for this field. We have found out what is going on in alcoholic liver disease, but there may be other areas where glucagon may be of importance at this moment in research. Would anybody care to make any extra comments?

Fehér I am convinced of the beneficial effect of glucagon/insulin therapy in the severe toxic liver lesion on the basis of experimental and clinical data. That is why I should like to interrupt the controlled multicentric study in cases of alcoholic liver lesions with glucagon/insulin therapy and continue instead with the investigation of the treatment of alcoholic intoxication, in carbon tetrachloride intoxication, and also in mushroom intoxication. I am also of the opinion that further animal experiments and *in vitro* experiments with lymphocytes, granulocytes and hepatocytes are necessary in order to know the mechanism of action of glucagon/insulin in liver protection as well as in liver regeneration and also in the influence of lymphocytes and granulocytes interaction.

Oka I would like to add that I think glucagon is acting not only to stimulate regeneration of the liver but that it may also act to prevent liver injury. I agree with Professor Fehér's opinion.

Vilardell Any other comments?

Nikolov Well, let me say that I found the morning general discussion was quite straightforward because a lot of work has been done in the gastrointestinal and biliary systems with glucagon, and I do not think that we have so many questions to solve there. I think many things have already been clarified in the morning presentations but, in my opinion, the afternoon papers give rise to many questions which would require not only more extensive *in vitro* and *in vivo* studies in order to further investigate the possible mechanisms of action of glucagon and insulin as hepatotrophics, but also more comprehensive clinical data both on toxically- and viral-induced acute liver necrosis. I would even go as far as suggesting that this topic alone deserves for itself a meeting such as this one some years from now.

Vilardell So it seems we are bound to have a fourth meeting on glucagon in three or four years!

Baker I think this line of discussion raises the difficult question that you get into in clinical medicine as to how many studies you need before you consider a new therapy established, and I do not know what the answer is, I do not know if it is three or four, but for my judgement it is more than one. For that reason, even though I am enthusiastic about the possibilities of insulin and glucagon for alcoholic hepatitis, we do not use it yet in our hospital in an uncontrolled fashion, we still enter patients into this same study which you have just heard about, despite Professor Fehér's results. I dare say that if I had achieved his results, then we would be giving insulin and glucagon to the patients in our hospital. But I certainly think that for the generalized acceptance of insulin/glucagon therapy for alcoholic hepatitis we are going to need more than one controlled study to show that it is beneficial, which means that we need additional patient studies in this connection, and you could say the same thing about fulminant hepatic failure which to me, and I think to most people in most parts of the world with the exception of Japan, means that we need to know what effect we are having on mortality, and here again I think there is room for additional studies looking at the most severely ill patients with fulminant hepatic failure for which the only treatment now, which has only been a fact since the last year or two, would be liver transplantation, where it is available. These patients can be transplanted effectively, but it is an expensive, high cost type of procedure, and if glucagon and insulin were clearly beneficial, it is obvious that this would be the best way to go. However, I think we need more animal studies as well because we have got to understand, in the way that Dr Fujiwara has tried to do, what the mechanism of any effect on hepatic regeneration is, what the intrahepatic effects of these hormones are and whether there are, indeed, other substances which may be important. So I am quite sure that in about five years there is going to be plenty of data for another conference which I believe by then can be devoted solely to liver regeneration.

Vilardell   I am very glad to see that we have all reached the same conclusion in this point.

Remarks from the chairmen

At this moment the day's sessions had to be called to an end in spite of ourselves, for, as can be imagined, we could have gone on for hours. As on previous occasions this workshop had proved to be very informative and rewarding, and tired as we naturally were, we were also refreshed and satisfied.

We who have had the opportunity to attend the previous meetings on glucagon felt a particular satisfaction at seeing our wishes for a third workshop materialize, and though much has been said already in favour of this type of meeting, on this occasion too we realized that it is not only the challenge of laying out and discussing so much in such a short time that is important. It proved to be just as stimulating to be among people gathered from very different nationalities and cultures and share their interests and opinions far beyond the scientific level or the limitations of language and culture. We can only be grateful that communications have not yet become too 'technified'; people are still forced to move around to meet each other personally. On occasions such as this one cannot help feeling that the day will come when we will be able to participate in a meeting such as this but without moving from our homes and that indeed then a very valuable asset will have been lost.

We are confident that the publication of the proceedings of this workshop, not only will enable you, the reader, to partake of the information and points of view that were raised and discussed, but will incite you, by reading through this book, to express your own opinions or experiences, place new questions or add further information, so that this will not be just the end result of a meeting that took place some time ago, but a starting point for an on-going colloquy. To make this possible, at the beginning of the book you will find the addresses of all the participants of this workshop who will be more than pleased to hear from you.

A. ORIOL-BOSCH
F. VILARDELL

Index

A-cells, glucagon synthesis 4
acetoacetate 6
acetylcholine 26
adenosine monophosphate *see* cyclic AMP
    (adenosine monophosphate)
adenylase 6
adenylate cyclase 15–16
adipose cells, effect of glucagon 6, 9
adrenaline 16
α-adrenergic antagonists, effect on sphincter
    of Oddi 76
β-adrenergic antagonists, effect on sphincter
    of Oddi 76
albumin, levels in acute hepatitis 128
alcohol
    consumption 111, 112
    intoxication 165
    'safe' daily limits 111
alcoholic hepatitis 165
    alcohol intake of study groups 114
    with cirrhosis 122
    glucagon and insulin therapy 113–21,
        165–6
        acute hepatitis response
            compared 133
        comparison of studies 119
        controlled trials 152–4
        results 116
        studied together and separately 123
        survival rate 123
    hepatic blood flow 160
    incidence 111
    sex differences in disturbance of liver
        function 114, 120

survival rates 152, 153
symptoms 112
treatment 112
amino-acids
    branched chain 141
    circulatory pattern of, in plasma 7
    in glucagonoma 94
    in hepatic regeneration 147, 148
    sequence in various species 3
AMP (adenosine monophosphate) *see* cyclic
    AMP (adenosine monophosphate)
antibiotics 141, 142
antibodies, inhibiting glucagon
    secretion 12
anticholinergics 164
    animal studies of bile secretion 68
    compared with glucagon in
        radiology 29, 31–4
        relative costs 34
    contraindications 30
        glaucoma 55
        prostatic hypertrophy 55, 64
    effect in oesophageal hypotonia 89–90
    endoscopic retrograde cholangio-
        pancreatography (ERCP) 80
    premedication for endoscopy 55
    in radiology, deaths 38–9
    side-effects in radiology 29–30, 32–4
antithrombin III 141
appetite regulation 13
atropine
    effect on sphincter of Oddi 76
    in radiology 41
    use with glucagon 90

atropine sulphate, use in upper gastrointestinal tract radiology   35–6, 38

barium enema
coating of mucosa   30, 31–2
double contrast
diagnostic accuracy compared with
single contrast   45–7
indications   42
retrograde ileography   47
sensitivity reactions   42, 45
spasm decreased by glucagon   47
use of CO_2 instead of air   47
premedication   164
bile, composition during glucagon
infusion   92
bile duct, pressures   75
bile flow, related to splanchnic blood
flow   91–2
bile secretion
mechanisms   68
role of glucagon
animal studies   68
human studies   68–9
biliary disorders
cholecystography   78
colic, therapy   164
intravenous infusion
cholangiography   79
operative cholangiography and
radiomanometry   79
pain relieved by glucagon   80
percutaneous transhepatic cholangiography   79
postoperative concretions   85
ultrasound investigation   78
bilirubin
effect of glucagon   84
levels in acute hepatitis   128
blood
circulation, effect of glucagon   16–17, 92
coagulation, therapy   141
brain, glucagon levels   13
brain oedema, therapy   141
butropium bromide   38
endoscopic retrograde cholangiography
(ERCP)   80
side effects   32–4

calcitonin, stimulated by glucagon   13

calcium, in hepatic regeneration   147, 148
calcium metabolism   13, 122
cancers
colo-rectal, use of computed
tomography   49
hepatocellular   112
carbon dioxide, substitution for air in
radiography   47
carbon tetrachloride intoxication   165
carnitine transferase   6
catecholamine release   7, 17
catheters, introduction   65
children, intramuscular administration of
glucagon   90
cholangiography
endoscopic retrograde   57–8, 80, 164
intravenous infusion   79
operative   79
percutaneous transhepatic   79
cholecystectomy, effect of glucagon on bile
secretion   68
cholecystography, biliary disorders   78
choledocholithiasis, use of glucagon   80
choleretic effect of glucagon   81, 164
cholesterol
circulating levels   7
excretion   92
levels in acute hepatitis   128
cirrhosis see liver, cirrhosis
colchicine, alcoholic hepatitis therapy   112
Coliopan (butropium bromide), side-
effects   32–4
colitis   47
colon, motility, effect of glucagon   81–3, 84
colonoscopy, premedication   164
computed tomography, colo-rectal
cancers   49
corticosteroids
alcoholic hepatitis therapy   112
in hepatic regeneration   149
cortisol   9
Crohn's disease   47, 163–4
cyclic AMP (adenosine
monophosphate)   26
glucagon blocking agents   12
levels increased by adenylate cyclase
activation   16
production   6
cystic fibrosis, biliary concretions   85
cytochrome P450 activation   108

dehistidine glucagon   12
diabetics
    effect of glucagon in endoscopy   53
    glucagon ineffective in gastrointestinal
        radiology   52–3
    and glucagonoma   94
    use of pump to deliver glucagon   85–6
diclofenac   164
diuretics   141
diverticulitis   47
DNA (deoxyribonucleic acid), accelerated
    synthesis with glucagon and
    insulin   100, 106
duodenography   163
    value of glucagon   41
duodenum, intraluminal pressures   58–9, 75

encephalopathy, hepatic
    with alcoholic hepatitis   114–15
    therapy   141
endoscopic manometry, sphincter of
    Oddi   71–2
endoscopic retrograde cholangio-
    pancreatography (ERCP)   164
    biliary disorders   80
    premedication   57–8
endoscopy
    digestive tract, glucagon in
        premedication   55–63
    and effect of glucagon in diabetics   53
    upper gastrointestinal tract
        glucagon as premedication   56
        side-effects of premedication   34
epidermal growth factor   107
    binding to hepatocyte membranes   150
    in hepatic regeneration   133, 147, 148,
        150
    hepatocyte proliferation   148, 150
epinephine   9, 12
exercise, stimulating glucagon release   8, 9,
    12–13

α-fetoprotein
    levels in acute hepatitis   128, 131
    market of liver regeneration   133
fibroblast growth factor   107
    and liver regeneration   157, 158
free fatty acids (FFA)   6
    levels in diabetics   52
fulminant hepatitis   132–3, 166

available therapies   140–2
blood exchange   138, 144
causes of death   140
diagnosis   136
glucagon and insulin therapy   135–43,
    154
    administration   136
    clinical evaluation   136–40
    ethical considerations   144–5
    therapeutic effect   137–9
    hypoglycaemia   145, 154
    length of survival period   139
    mortality rate   135
    prednisolone therapy   136, 137–8, 143
    survival rate   136, 138–9, 140
    related to therapy mode   142

gallbladder motility   69
    effect of glucagon   69, 71
gastric acid secretion inhibition
    by glucagon   90
    by oxyntomodulin   6
    for radiology   38
gastric juice secretion
    problems   91
    use of atropine   90
gastrointestinal endoscopy, side-effects of
    premedication   34
gastrointestinal radiology, without
    premedication   34
gastrointestinal tract
    bleeding, therapy   141
    effect of glucagon on smooth muscle   89
    radiology, uses of glucagon   162–3
    see also lower gastrointestinal tract: upper
        gastrointestinal tract
glaucoma
    anticholergenics contraindicated   55
    use of glucagon   64
glicentin   5
glicentin-related pancreatic peptide
    (GRPP)   5
glucagon
    acute hepatitis therapy   125–31
    alcholic hepatitis therapy   113–21
    animal studies extrapolated to man   94
    binding to hepatocyte membranes   150
    compared with anticholinergics in
        radiography   29, 31–4
        relative costs   34

glucagon (*continued*)
    compared with anticholinergics in
        gastrointestinal radiography   41
    control of release   7–8
    counter-regulatory role   8–9
    digestive endoscopy, premedi-
        cation   55–63
    dosage rate
        effect on bile and bile components   84
        in radiology   38
        physiological and pharmacological
            effects 67
    effect of intermittent administration   89
    effect of mixed meal   93
    effect of smooth muscle in gastrointestinal
        tract   89
    effectiveness in liver failure   103–5
    endoscopic retrograde cholangio-
        pancreatography (ERCP)   57–8
        compared with prifinium bromide   59
        limitations on use   63
    evanescent effect   88
    as free-radical scavenger   122
    fulminant hepatitis therapy   135–43
    in hepatic regeneration   147–8
    hepatotrophic effect   99–106
    inhibition by antibodies   12
    intra-islet release, related to insulin and
        somatostatin release   8
    intramuscular administration, in
        children   90
    levels in diabetics   52
    in lower gastrointestinal
        radiography   41–9
        cases where ineffective   52–3
        and diagnostic accuracy   46
        dose rate   52
    mechanism of liver protection   165
    mode of action   17
    molecular weight   3
    pharmacological action   76
    physiological effects   6–7
        sphincter of Oddi   73, 75
    primary structure   3
    production by genetic engineering   37
    ratio to insulin   6
    receptors *see* receptors
    regulation   16
    relationship with biliary tree   67
    restoration of hepatocyte function   103
    role in hepatocyte proliferation   100
    secretion *see* secretion
    sensitivity reactions with barium
        enema   45
    species difference in effects   84–5
    synthesis *see* synthesis
    in upper gastrointestinal tract
        radiology   29–36
glucagonoma   94
glucose
    effect of glucagon on output   88
    homeostasis
        controlled by liver   8
        neonatal   9
    oscillating secretion   89
    output increased by glucagon   6
glycerin   141
glycogenolytic effect   6, 16
glycylhistidyllysine   149
growth hormone   9
GTP   16
gut glucagon-like immunoreactive materials
    (GLIs)   5

H_2-receptor antagonists   141, 142
heart, effects of glucagon   7
hepatic encephalopathy
    with alcoholic hepatitis   114–15
    therapy   141
hepatic regeneration *see* liver, regeneration
hepatitis
    acute, glucagon and insulin
        therapy   125–31
        alcoholic hepatitis response
            compared   133
        results of study   127
        serum transaminase levels   127
    alcoholic *see* alcoholic hepatitis
    fulminant *see* fulminant hepatitis
    viral   126
        glucagon and insulin therapy   120
hepatocytes
    appearance in alcoholic hepatitis   114
    binding of circulating growth
        factors   150–1
    grain tracks on membrane   18
    location of receptors   15
    necrosis, therapy   141
    proliferation
        intracellular signals   151

hepatocytes (*continued*)
  proliferation (*continued*)
    role of epidermal growth factor   148
    role of glucagon and insulin   100
  restoration of function   103
  role of glucagon in ultrastructural
      modification   17
  target cells of glucagon   6
  transport of bile acids   68
  see also liver
histamine, vasodilating effect   16
hormones, role in metabolism   15
β-hydroxybutyrate   6
hyoscine, endoscopic retrograde cholangio-
    pancreatography (ERCP)   80
hyoscine butylbromide   38
hyperaminoacidaemia, stimulating glucagon
    release   8
hyperbilirubinaemia
  in alcoholic hepatitis   112
  postoperative, glucagon infusion   91
  reduction   81
hypergammaglobulinaemia, in alcoholic
    hepatitis   112
hyperglycaemia   88
  inhibiting glucagon release   8
hyperinsulinaemia, inhibiting glucagon
    release   8
hypo-albuminaemia, in alcoholic
    hepatitis   112
hypocalcaemia, effects of glucagon
    therapy   13
hypoglycaemia   45, 105
  acute hepatitis   127
  alcoholic hepatitis   116
  fulminant hepatitis   145, 154
  glucagon first line of defence   9
  stimulating glucagon release   8, 9

ileal plugs   47
infections, therapy   141
inflammatory bowel disease, detection   45,
    46
insulin
  acute hepatitis therapy   125–31
  alcholic hepatitis therapy   113–21
  binding to hepatocyte membranes   150
  effectiveness in liver failure   103–5
  fulminant hepatitis therapy   135–43
  in hepatic regeneration   147–8

hepatotrophic effect   99–106
intra-islet release, related to glucagon and
    somatostatin release   8
  mechanism of liver protection   165
  oscillating secretion   87
  pulsatile secretion   89
  ratio to glucagon   6
  restoration of hepatocyte function   103
  role in hepatocyte proliferation   100
  stimulating release   7
intravenous infusion cholangiography, biliary
    disorders   79
intussusception, reduction   47–9
iotroxamide, secretion enhanced by
    glucagon   92
islets of Langerhans, pattern of hormone
    release   8

ketogenesis   6
ketone bodies   6
  levels in diabetics   52
kidneys
  effects of glucagon   7
  failure, therapy   141

L-cells, production of glicentin   5
lactulose   141
leukocytes, glucagoneric receptors   17
lipolytic effect   6, 9, 16
liver
  cirrhosis   111, 112
    alcohol consumption levels   111
    in alcoholic hepatitis   114, 122
  disease
    glucagon and insulin therapy, controlled
        trials   152–4
    inhibited by glucagon and insulin   120
    related to alcohol consumption
        111–12
    severity in women   120
    types due to alcohol   112
    see also hepatitis
  failure
    effectiveness of glucagon and
        insulin   99, 100, 103–5
    fulminant   125, 132–3
  fatty   112
  homogenates, in hepatic regeneration
      149
  protein content levels   102
  receptor sites   25

liver (*continued*)
  recovery from injury   102
  regeneration   147–55, 166
    in animals   147–9
    binding of circulating growth factors
      150–1
    ethical considerations of studies   158
    fields for future studies   155, 159
    in humans   151–2
    importance of blood supply   147–8,
      152
    interaction of factors   149–50
    partial hepatectomy of rat models   107
    role of epidermal growth factor   135
    stimulator substances   149
    studies in toxically induced damage and
      partial hepatectomy   157–8
  toxically and virally induced
    necrosis   165
  see also hepatocytes
lower gastrointestinal tract
  colonic motility, effect of glucagon   61–3,
    64
  radiology   163, 164
  use of glucagon   41–9

malonyl-CoA   6
mannitol   141
meconium ileus   47
metabolism, role of hormones   15
metoclopramide, increased intra-oesophageal
  and gastric pressures   57
morphine
  effect on gastrointestinal motility,
    compared with glucagon   76, 85
  in radiology   41
mushroom intoxication   165
myorelaxant action   18, 24, 26

N (regulating protein)   16
naloxone, and spasm in sphincter of
  Oddi   85
neoglycogenesis   16
neonatal effects of glucagon   9
neonatal hyperbilirubinaemia   81
neoplasms, detection   45, 46
neostigmine, effect on colonic motility   62
neurones, intestinal nervous plexuses,
  glucagon receptors   24–5
noradrenaline   16
  vasoconstrictive effect   16

oesophageal difuse spasm   65
oesophageal disorders, role of glucagon
  162
oesophageal hypotonia, anticholinergics
  89–90
oesophageal manometry   65
oesophogastric manometry, use of
  glucagon   56–7
operative cholangiography, biliary
  disorders   79
oxyntomodulin   5, 6
  inhibition of gastric acids   38

pancreas, pressures   75
pancreatitis, effect of glucagon on
  pressure   93–4
papaverine   18
papilla of Vater, intraluminal pressures   58–9
D-penicillamine, alcoholic hepatitis
  therapy   112
pentolinium, effect on sphincter of Oddi   76
percutaneous transhepatic cholangiography,
  biliary disorders   79
phaeochromocytoma   7, 45
  radiology utilising glucagon   37
pharmacological action of glucagon   76
phenoxybenzamine, effect on sphincter of
  Oddi   76
phosphodiesterases
  inhibitors   18
  regulating glucagon action   16
plasmapheresis   139, 141, 144
platelet growth factor, and liver
  regeneration   157, 158
pneumocolon examination, peroral   49
polyps, detection   45, 46
portal hypertension, hepatic blood flow
  160
prednisolone, fulminant hepatitis
  therapy   136, 137–8, 143
preproglucagon   4
prifinium bromide, compared with glucagon,
  in endoscopic retrograde
  cholangiopancreatography   59
proglucagon   4–5
propantheline bromide, in radiology   41
propranolol
  effect on portal pressure   92
  effect on sphincter of Oddi   76
prostaglandin E_2, vasodilating effect   16

prostaglandins, in hepatic regeneration 149, 150
prostatic hypertrophy
  anticholergenics contraindicated 55, 64
  use of glucagon 64

radiography
  double-contrast techniques 34
  effect of glucagon, as bolus 76
  premedication, sequence 34–6
radiology
  lower intestinal tract, use of glucagon 41–9
  premedication 29, 30
  upper gastrointestinal tract, role of glucagon 29–36
  use of double-contrast techniques 29
  see also barium enema
radiomanometry, biliary disorders 79
receptors 6, 15
  action of glucagon on 25–6
  location 18, 20, 23
    on hepatocytes 15
  quantification 20
  turnover, replacement and generation 87
retrograde ileography 47

saline, in endoscopic retrograde cholangiopancreatography (ERCP) 80
sclerosing cholangitis, need to void bile plugs 86
secretin infusion 141
secretion
  oscillating 87
  pattern 87–9
  pulsatile 87, 88
silibinin, alcoholic hepatitis therapy 112
small intestine
  glucagon activity 18, 20, 24
  radiology 163
  retrograde ileography 47
smooth muscle
  effect of glucagon 7, 17, 25, 76
    gastrointestinal tract 89
    intravenous or intramuscular 55

somatostatin
  animal studies of bile secretion 68
  intra-islet release, related to glucagon and somatostatin release 8
spasmolytic effect 18, 25
sphincter of Oddi
  effect of glucagon on motility and pressure 57–8
  effects of α- and β-adrenergic antagonists 76
  endoscopic manometry 71–2
  motility 71
  physiological effects of glucagon 73, 75
  pressures 71–2
  relaxation 93
  structure and function 71
starvation, stimulating glucagon release 9
stress, stimulating glucagon release 8, 9
synthesis of glucagon
  fragment assembly 3–4
  in vitro 3
  location 4
  sites 13
  stepwise assembly 4

theophylline 18
thrombocyte growth factor 107
thyroid hormone, in hepatic regeneration 147, 148
triglycerides, circulating levels 7

ultrasound investigation, biliary disorders 78
upper gastrointestinal tract
  endoscopy, glucagon as premedication 56
  role of glucagon in radiology 29–36

vagal system stimulation, stimulating glucagon release 8
vascular system, effect of glucagon 25
vasoactive action 15
vasodilatory effects 15, 16
viral hepatitis 126
  glucagon and insulin therapy 120

women, severity of alcohol-induced liver disease 114, 120